JOHN EBNEZAR **CBS** | Handbooks i
Orthope

SERIES

Practical Examination

Viva Voce in

Practical Orthopedic Examination

VOLUME II

- Splints and Plasters
- Traction in Orthopedics
- Prosthetics and Orthotics
- Specimen and Slides
- Spotters

to

my mother (late) Sampath Kumari

my wife Dr Parimala

my lovely children Rakesh and Priyanka

and

all my patients

John Ebnezar —————————————————————

- Holder of the **Guinness Book of World Records** for the most number of books written by an individual in a single year.
- Listed in the **India Book of Records** for the most number of books written by an individual.
- Recipient of the highest civilian awards of Karnataka, the **Rajyotsava Award 2010** and the **Kempegowda Award 2011**.
- Recipient of the **Best Citizen of India Award** by the International Publishing house.
- Former Vice-President, the Indian Orthopaedic Association
- President, Neuro-Spinal Surgeons Association of India (Karnataka)
- CEO, Parimala Health Care Services, A ISO 9001:2008 Hospital, Bilekahalli, Bannerghatta Road, Bangalore
- Ebnezar Orthopedic Center, Bilekahalli, Bannerghatta Road, Bangalore
- Dr John's Orthopedic Clinic, near Reliance Mart, Arakere, BG Road, Bangalore
- Chairman, the Physically Handicapped and Paraplegic Charitable Trust of Karnataka®
- Founder President, Geriatric Orthopedic Society
- Founder President, Orthopedic Authors Association and All India Medical Authors Association
- Chairman, Karnataka Orthopedic Academy®
- President, Bangalore Holistic Academy
- Chairman, Rakesh Cultural Academy
- President, Vaidya Kala Ranga, Bangalore
- Secretary, SK Educational Society®
- Former Senior Specialist, Victoria Hospital, Bangalore Medical College, Bangalore
- Former Assistant Professor in Orthopedics, Devaraj Urs Medical College, Kolar, Karnataka
- Postgraduate teacher, Bangalore Baptist Hospital, Airport Road, Bangalore

JOHN EBNEZAR **CBS** | Handbooks in
Orthopedics and Fractures

SERIES —————————————————————————————————

Practical Examination

Viva Voce in
Practical Orthopedic
Examination

VOLUME II

- Splints and Plasters
- Traction in Orthopedics
- Prosthetics and Orthotics
- Specimen and Slides
- Spotters

John Ebnezar

MBBS, D'Ortho, DNB (Ortho), MNAMS (Ortho), PhD (Yoga)
Sports Medicine (Australia), INOR Fellow (UK), DAc, DMT

Consulting Orthopedic and Spine Surgeon
Holistic Orthopedic Expert, and Sports Specialist
Bangalore

CBS Publishers & Distributors Pvt Ltd
New Delhi • Bengaluru • Pune • Kochi • Chennai

Disclaimer
Science and technology are constantly changing
fields. New research and experience broaden the
scope of information and knowledge. The author has
tried his best in giving information available to him
while preparing the material for this book. Although,
all efforts have been made to ensure optimum
accuracy of the material, yet it is quite possible some
errors might have been left uncorrected. The publisher,
printer and author will not be held responsible for any
inadvertent errors or inaccuracies.

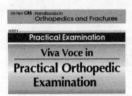

ISBN: 978-81-239-2151-8

Copyright © Author and Publisher

First Edition: 2012

All rights reserved. No part of this book may be reproduced or
transmitted in any form or by any means, electronic or
mechanical, including photocopying, recording, or any
information storage and retrieval system without permission, in
writing, from the author and the publisher.

Published by Satish Kumar Jain and produced by Vinod K. Jain for
CBS Publishers & Distributors Pvt Ltd
4819/XI Prahlad Street, 24 Ansari Road, Daryaganj
New Delhi 110 002, India.   Website: www.cbspd.com
Ph: 23289259, 23266861, 23266867   e-mail: delhi@cbspd.com
Fax: 011-23243014   cbspubs@airtelmail.in.

Branches

- Bengaluru: Seema House 2975, 17th Cross, K.R. Road,
  Banasankari 2nd Stage, Bengaluru 560 070, Karnataka
  Ph: +91-80-26771678/79   Fax: +91-80-26771680   e-mail: bangalore@cbspd.com

- Pune: Bhuruk Prestige, Sr. No. 52/12/2+1+3/2 Narhe, Haveli
  (Near Katraj-Dehu Road Bypass), Pune 411 051, Maharashtra
  Ph: 020-64704058, 64704059, 32392277 Fax: +91-020-24300160 e-mail: pune@cbspd.com

- Kochi: 36/14 Kalluvilakam, Lissie Hospital Road, Kochi 682 018,
  Kerala
  Ph: +91-484-4059061-65   Fax: +91-484-4059065   e-mail: cochin@cbspd.com

- Chennai: 20, West Park Road, Shenoy Nagar, Chennai 600 030,
  Tamil Nadu
  Ph: +91-44-26260666, 26208620   Fax: +91-44-45530020   email: chennai@cbspd.com

Printed at Magic International, Greater Noida (UP)

Preface

As a student of orthopedics, I enjoyed the experience of the studentship. Practical examination in our life as a student is always going to be an acid test. It was a mountain which every student wanted to scale successfully. The complexity of the practical examination made us run around the wards, journal clubs, libraries, rehabilitation departments, X-ray centers and to pathology department. We used to attend seminars, group discussions and special lecture classes. We used to grasp as much as possible because we would always fall short of expectations in practical examinations. As the final exams approach, we panic. We build into small groups for discussions and run around the wards seeing as many cases as possible not knowing what cases will be given. Unfortunately, we never got to see all the cases shown in the exams at one go or got to see the X-rays all at a time, or the instruments and implants all assembled as a single unit, or had sufficient time to go to the pathology department to see the specimen and slides.

As a DNB student, the situation was far worse as the centers of practical exams were alien and the atmosphere unfamiliar. There was no way we could revise the practical formats. It was at this time I felt if there ever was a book that deals all practical examination from cases to orthotics, then it would have made my life easy during the crucial hours of practical exams.

Also, such a book could give us an opportunity for us to revise and repeatedly to our satisfaction. And if the book could give us the most likely questions that would be asked in the practical exams, then it would be still better as we would now know what to concentrate upon and what the examiner expects from us.

During practical exams, I have noticed students frantically looking for clues, for diagnosis, they try to peep into the X-rays, case papers, etc. They keep pleading with the seniors, experts, medical students, staff, attendees and even patients for some vital information. To my chagrin, many times I have seen students being misguided by wrong leads or suggestions even though they had made the right diagnosis. I have seen the best of students not succeeding in practical exams.

It was then I decided to write a book that caters to practical examination in its entirety. What was presumed to be a fairly simple journey, turned out to be the most arduous one? Now, the book is complete and is before you. I have tried my best to include all aspects of practical examinations. But putting everything in one book increased the size of the book and a student may not be interested to know everything and may be interested to know about certain isolated aspect of the practical examination. Hence a series of books concerning all aspects of practical examination in orthopedics is brought out. This is useful for the postgraduate students in orthopedics, undergraduate students and also the examiners.

I have divided various aspects of Viva Voce Section of the practical examination into two volumes. Volume I of this book deals with important aspect of practical viva voce examination like the typical X-rays, instruments and implants, as well as common orthopedic surgeries that are usually asked in the practical examinations. And the rest part of the viva voce examination comprising splints and plasters, traction, prosthetics and orthotics, specimen and slides and spotters is included in this Volume II and I have taken care to include most of the information but some of the matter may still be missing. This book aims to give you an insight into what happens and what you should do during the Viva Voce in the exams. It acts as a guide but ultimately it is up to you to perform, keeping the information given in this book in the back of your mind. In case you want to know about other aspects of the viva voce section of the practical examination, I suggest you to read Volume I of this series.

But I know, despite my best efforts there would be inadequate, unnecessary or missing information. This is due to different requirements by the universities across the country. I request the students to please ignore these minor blemishes. I will be happy if the students find this book useful and helpful during the practical exams. Feedback will be valued.

John Ebnezar

Acknowledgments

This volume is a part of the 100⁺ book series brought out in a single calendar year. This was a huge and mammoth task attempted first time ever by an author and a publisher in the world. Such an herculean effort could not have been possible without the active involvement of those concerned in CBS Publishers & Distributors. I thank Mr Satish K Jain, Managing Director of CBS P&D, for agreeing to be a part of this world-record feat in bringing out this book in the Series. My special thanks to Mr YN Arjuna who showed special interest in this work and channelized his entire energy into this improbable feat. My special thanks to Mrs Ritu Chawla and her entire dedicated team who have toiled day and night to make this dream a reality. I thank members of the entire editorial–production team of CBS P&D who have worked hard behind the scenes to bring out this book.

My special thanks to Dr Yogitha for actively helping me in the compilation of all the books. I also thank all the staff members of my hospital who have helped me at various levels during the making of this book.

John Ebnezar

Contents

4. Specimen and Slides 78

TITLES IN THE SERIES

I Orthopedic Trauma

II Orthopedic Disease

III Specific Orthopedic Problems

IV Regional Orthopedic Problems

V Orthopedic Injuries and Surgeries

Upper Limb

Lower Limb

IX Yoga Therapy in Common Orthopedic Problems

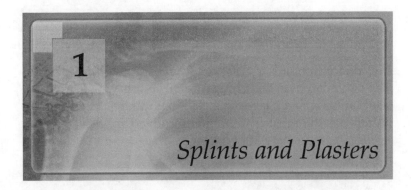

Splints and Plasters

Splints and plasters are important methodology of treatment in orthopedics. Splints are mainly used as a firstaid measure to immoblize the fractures before definitive treatment. Plasters on the other hand could be used as a temporary or permanent method of treatment of fractures. This book deals with important splints and plasters in orthopaedics and is useful to the students as well as general readers.

Splints in Orthopedics
- Plaster of Paris splints
- Factors influencing plastering

Functional Cast Brace
- Mode of action

Important Splints in Orthopedics other than POP
- Thomas splint
- Böhler-Braun (BB) splint

Let us begin with the most likely questions that will be asked in the viva voce.

SPLINTS IN ORTHOPEDICS

1. What is a splint and what forms a splint?
Ans. Any material which is used to support a fracture is called a splint. From a folded newspaper, wood, cardboard, etc. to the present-day thermoplastics anything can act as a splint. The former is called an unconventional splint and is

used more as an improvisation splints in carrying out the first aid for fractures in emergency where things are not ideal. The latter can be called conventional splints which are more sophisticated and effective. In orthopedic practice POP splints are the most commonly employed splints.

Remember
- Anything acts as a splint including ones own uninjured part of the body.
- Splint is a material used to support fractures.
- Unconventional splints are crude, temporary and are used as a first aid measure, e.g. book, paper, umbrella, wood, etc.
- Conventional splints are refined sophisticated and serve both as first aid and definitive measures, e.g. POP splint, Thomas splint, Böholer-Braun splint, etc.

To attain the goal of fracture treatment of restoring anatomy to normal, splints help a long way. They form the mainstay of conservative treatment of fractures.

PLASTER OF PARIS SPLINTS

Must Know Facts

2. Do you know the interesting history behind the name plaster of Paris?

Ans. The name plaster of Paris originated from an accident to a house built on deposit of gypsum near the city of Paris. The house was accidentally burnt down. When it rained on the next day, it was noted that the footprints of the people in the mud had set rock hard. Plaster of Paris was first used in orthopedics by Mathysen, a Dutch surgeon, in 1852. It is made from gypsum which is a naturally occurring mineral. It is commercially available since 1931.

Chemical Formula

3. Name the chemical formula of plaster of Paris.

Ans. It is a hemihydrated calcium sulphate. To make plaster of Paris, gypsum is heated to drive off water. When water is added to the resulting powder original mineral forms and is set hard.

$$2(CaSO_4 \cdot 2H_2O) + Heat \Leftrightarrow 2(CaSO_4 \cdot \frac{1}{2}H_2O) + 3H_2O$$

POP Types

4. What are the types of POP?

Ans. Two types of POP are in usage.

Indigenous

Prepared from ordinary cotton bandage role smeared with POP powder.

Commercial

Plaster of Paris rolls commercially prepared consists of rolls of muslin stiffened by starch POP power and an accelerator substance like alum. This commercial preparation sets very fast gives a neat finish unlike the indigenous ones.

5. Why is plaster of Paris an ideal splint?

Ans.

- It is cheap
- It is easily available
- It is comfortable
- It is easy to mould
- It is quick setting
- It is strong and light
- It is easy to remove
- It is permeable to radiography
- It is permeable to air and hence underlying skin can breathe.
- It is non-inflammable.

Various Forms

6. What are the various forms of POP?

Ans. Plaster of Paris is used in four forms as slab, cast, spica and functional cast brace.

Slab

7. What is a slab? Name the different methods.

Ans. It is a temporary splint used in the initial stages of fracture treatment and also during first aid. It is useful to immobilize the limbs postoperatively and in infections. It is made up of half by POP and half by bandage roll and hence can accommodate the swelling in the initial stages of fractures. Slab is prepared according to the required length. There are three methods of applying a slab.

Dry method: Here the slab is prepared first and then dipped in water (commonly employed).

Wet method: Here the slab is prepared after dipping the POP roll in water. This is rare and requires experience.

Pattern method: Here the slabs are fashioned in the desired way before dipping it in water.

Casts

8. What is a cast? Name the different methods.

Ans. Here the POP roll completely encircles the limb. It is used as a definitive form of fracture treatment and also to correct deformities. There are three methods of applying a POP cast.

Skin tight cast: Here the cast is directly applied over the skin. Dangerous as it may cause pressure sores. It is difficult to remove as the hairs may be incorporated into the cast and hence it is not recommended.

Bologna cast: Here generous amount of cotton padding is applied to the limb before putting the cast. This is the commonly employed method.

Three-tier cast: Here stockinette is used first over which cotton padding is done before applying the POP cast. It is an ideal method, but it is expensive.

Spica

9. Define a spica.

Ans. Spica encircles a part of the body, e.g. hip spica for fracture around the hip, thumb spica for fracture scaphoid.

Functional Cast Brace

10. What is a functional cast brace?

Ans. Functional cast brace is used for fracture tibia after initial immobilization of 3 to 4 weeks.

11. Name the important issues relating to a plaster.

Ans.

• Factors influencing plastering.
• Preparation of the patients.
• Plaster application principles.
• Care of the cast.
• Instructions to patients.
• Complications.
• Removal of plaster casts.

Factors Influencing Plastering

12. What are the factors influencing plastering?

Ans. Although plaster of Paris only depends on one simple chemical reaction for its setting, it is possible to vary the features of the process according to different requirements.

Temperature

If a bandage is immersed in cold water the initial set will be delayed and thus working time lengthened. However, if a very rapid set is required, soaking the bandage in warm water will accelerate the rate of reaction. However, over 50°C, the setting rate slows and at 100°C no set occurs.

Strength

The final strength of the cast depends on the crystal structure. If the cast is manipulated after the initial set or prevented from drying out it will be weak. Drying out will be delayed in cold or moist conditions and accelerated in a warm and dry environment. Obviously, the cast strength is dependent upon the quality and thickness of plaster and the shape of the cast which follows the contours of the affected limb. However, excess plaster will also increase weight and bulk and heat released. Therefore, these different factors must be weighed against each other.

Padding

Padding is used under a plaster cast to mechanically protect the skin, soft tissue and bony abrasion during cast removal.

Padding is also necessary to protect the skin from thermal injury because of the exotherm generated during setting. Poorly applied padding may reproduce sores. Over padding will reduce the closeness of the fit of the cast and possibly permit excess movement at the fracture site resulting in impaired healing. Thus, skill in padding is as essential as plaster moulding in the production of a therapeutic cast.

Incorporation

Because plaster of Paris is infinitely mouldable in the wet state, it can be set around cast brace, hinges and walking heels with ease. However, for maximum strength the plaster should dry out first and the walking attachment should be affixed with a fresh plaster of bandage.

Absorption

Too much exudates from inside or moisture from outside the cast will reduce the strength of the cast and make it liable to breakdown.

Time

The strength of plaster of Paris builds up over a period of time and so load may be gradually increased. Excessive premature loading will produce a break down of the cast and patients need to be advised how much load they can apply and at what time.

Preparing for the Patient

13. What are the preparations for a patient?

Ans. Plaster casts are individually created for each patient. The clinical records of diagnosis and treatment may not always be available so prior to application of the cast it is essential to check that the right patient is receiving the right cast on the right part of the body.

Record

A record must be kept of each procedure with a note of the following:

- Personal details.
- Diagnosis and plaster type applied.
- Manipulation and anesthetic.
- Instructions given.
- Supplementary appliances given, e.g. crutches.
- Date of next attendance.

Some units record the name of the person who applied the cast. The last point is useful when trainee require supervision and guidance.

Any points to be noted particularly on a subsequent visit should be recorded.

Plaster Application Principles

14. Discuss the principles of plaster application.

Ans. The design and thickness of the cast must be appropriate to the kind of mechanical stresses which will be imposed on it. The amount of plaster applied depends upon the condition to be treated and the cast to which the cast will be put. Before padding or constructing a cast, it is imperative that the operator ensures that he has an adequate supply of materials and instruments within easy reach. Inadequate preparation can cause future cast weakness and breakdown.

Padding

15. What is the role of padding?

Ans. Soft material such as specialist orthopedic padding is placed on the skin before plaster application to prevent sores, to increase comfort and to act as a spacer to aid cast removal. Preferably, apply stockinette over the area to be plastered.

Unroll padding of the required width firmly over the area. Overlap each turn by one-third in order to secure the layers. If plaster slabs are to be incorporated in a padded cast, it is advisable to secure the padding with a complete layer of circular bandage that are applied under tension, wrinkling of the slab can occur. Padding is specially important in the following situations:

• When swelling is present or expected, i.e. in almost every acute condition.

• When the limb is thin and bones are very superficial.

• When electric plaster cutters are used for removal.

• When wedging is contemplated.

Application

Casts

16. Describe the technique of plaster cast application.

Ans. The following are the techniques of plaster cast application:

• With the equipment ready and either buckets or bowls filled with water (25–35°C), the patient is settled in a comfortable position with clothing protected. It is important that the patient is relaxed, comfortable and understands what is going to happen. If the patient is tense the finished cast can be loose and inefficient.

• The affected part should be covered with suitable padding and the desired position secured and held correctly. While maintaining the position the assistant hands must not obstruct the technician.

• Bandages of the correct size are immersed in water one at a time and held there until bubbling stops. The bandage is removed by holding it at the ends. The ends are gently squeezed towards the center then pulled back to shape. Wringing expels too much water and the bandage will become unworkable before application is complete and will not set properly.

- Keep the loading end free when handling the bandage to the operator. The operator unrolls the wet bandage around the limb in an even manner.

- Minimum tension should be exercised and this should be directed towards the center of the bandage and not at the edges.

- Only circular and spiral turns should be used. Reverse turns will lead to ridges inside the cast. Moulding of the bandages to the contours of the limb should be done by constant smoothing with the palms of the wet hands and by pleating at the upper or lower edges of the bandages, being careful to avoid bony prominences. Pleating will ensure that the central area of the bandage lies smoothly in the correct direction. Then tendency to build up a cast which is thick centrally and paper thin at the extremities can be prevented by making a double circular turn at the extremities.

- When the required thickness has been obtained the extremities of the cast may require trimming to ensure that a free range of movement is possible at joints which are not immobilized. This should be done while the cast is wet and not left until it is fully dried out. The completed wet cast is handled carefully and supported correctly to protect it from damage. The patient is suitably instructed in taking care of the casts.

Removable Splints

17. What are removable splints?

Ans. Plaster of Paris may be used for making removable splints. These fit the body part exactly.

Any complete cast can be converted into a removable splint by bivalving it. This is best done with an electric plaster cutter if the cast is padded. The edges of the cut remain firm and can be bound by bringing the stockinette over the edge and securing it with a strip of plaster bandage.

If a cast has been bivalved to facilitate daily dressing of a wound, and immobilization has to be continued, the anterior and posterior sections are both preserved and are held in place by a firm bandage.

Frequently, a removable splint to support the foot or wrist in the appropriate optimum position is requested. This can be achieved by the methods already described or a plaster slab to the required length and thickness is applied to the part while an assistant holds the joint in the desired position. This slab can be applied directly to the skin. It is carefully moulded, corners are trimmed and where necessary additional strengthening slabs can be positioned. Once set the cast can be trimmed and after removal the interior can be sprinkled with French chalk then polished with a pad of wool. This produces a light removable cast which is perfectly smooth and comfortable to wear. This cast requires to be dried out thoroughly before it is used by the patient.

Slabs

18. What is a slab? Describe the method of applications?
Slab is a temporary plaster of Paris splint that is used to support as injured or inflamed limb.
Ans. When the required length and width have been decided the slab is lightly folded from each end to the center. It is immersed in water, immediately removed then carefully and quickly smoothened on a flat surface. The layers must be pressed together and the bubble excluded. If this is not done the layers become brittle when dry and can separate giving an inefficient cast.

19. Name the methods of slab preparation.
Ans. Slabs can be prepared in two ways:
• By enrolling a GYPSONA bandage or bandages to a required length. This may be done with either wet or dry bandages which are folded out on a smooth surface. The average thickness of slabs for strengthening is five or six layers. When using bandages, care must be taken to see that all the layers extend for the same distance. Short ends should be discarded because they cannot be held securely

when the slab is immersed in water. Any inequality in length can cause a wrinkle or ridge to form.

- By withdrawing the required length of five layers thickness from a plaster slab pack or dispenser. This method is quicker and more reliable than the unrolling method.
- Slabs can be prepared in any width, depending on the need of the situation. Sometimes a slab is used for initial immobilization and is completed into a cast later. In this situation local pressure on the flesh at the edges can be eliminated if the layers are lightly "fanned" out from side to side. This adds to the patient's comfort and as the center retains its full thickness immobilization is not impaired in any way.
- Slabs must be smoothened carefully on a flat surface after they have been soaked. If this is not done the layers will be separated and the cast may become brittle.

Slabs for Strengthening Areas of Potential Weakness

20. Describe the role of slabs for strengthening areas of potential weakness.

Ans. Large joint areas such as the hip region need to be strengthened locally both anteriorly and posteriorly.

Where the pull of gravity is considerable as in the shoulder joint region, additional strengthening is desirable to prevent cracking and loss of position.

The margins of the body casts require additional strength to prevent softening which may be associated with handling and dampness when washing. Areas such as the sole of the foot which are subjected to considerable weight stresses and dampness from sweat need to be strengthened.

If a patient is obese, extra care must be taken to ensure that the cast is suitably reinforced.

21. Describe the use of slabs to reduce the overall weight of the cast.

Ans. This technique is applied to large casts particularly those that cover the trunk. For example, a plaster jacket can be made lighter and less bulky if slabs are applied over protective padding which has first been covered by a single layer of circular bandages as follows:

- Measured slabs should be placed along superior and inferior border.
- Measured slabs should be placed anteriorly from the sterna notch to the symphysis pubis and posteriorly from the upper border to the sacrum along the line of spine.
- Measured slabs should be placed laterally from the lower borders of the axillae to a point midway between the iliac crests and the greater trochanters.

Depending on the size of the patient, these slabs should be six or eight inches wide and of five layers thickness. If this procedure is followed encircling bandages are required only to secure the slabs. In this way both strength and lightness can be achieved.

Wet Cast

22. What is wet cast?

Ans. Freshly applied wet plaster of Paris casts become supportive in three to five minutes, depending on the water temperature and the thickness of the cast. The cast does not fully dry out until 36 to 72 hours after application. Examples of drying times:

- Forearm plaster: 36 hours.
- Leg plaster: 48 hours.
- Trunk plaster or plaster bed: 72 hours.

When a dry cast is tapped with the knuckles, it gives a crisp, clear sound, but the damp cast gives a dull sound.

Damage Due to Pressures

23. How to prevent damage of the cast due to pressure?

Ans. The supports used should be firm cushions which have a protective covering. A sheet or old towel should lie between the plaster and any waterproof surface. If this is not done, dampness will collect and cause softening of the plaster.

At home, the patient must be advised not to rest the wet cast on a firm surface such as an unpadded chair. This will dent the cast and produce a ridge on the internal surface which may cause soreness.

Drying Cast
24. What is a drying cast?
Ans. The most common method is to allow the cast to dry naturally in circulating air.

When possible the patients bed position should be changed every two to four hours to ensure even drying of both surfaces of the cast.

The out patient should be instructed to expose the cast to warm air but not to sit with one surface of the cast constantly directed towards heat (e.g. an electric heater).

Dry Cast
25. What are the instructions for a dry cast?
Ans. Once dry, the cast will tolerate moderate pressure but for walking a reinforcing sole or heel of wood or rubber should be added after the cast has dried.

Canvas or plastic coverings may be used for short periods to protect the cast from water. These must be removed regularly to prevent the plaster becoming damp as sweat fails to evaporate.

Forearm casts particularly are prone to getting wet at the lower edge which may fray. Small fragments may be detached and slip between the skin and plaster causing irritation. Thus, care of the cast is essential for healing without complications.

Instructions to Patients
26. What are the instructions to be given to all patients?
Ans. Written instructions should be given to all patients with plaster casts. Two examples are shown below.

All acute fracture casts should be checked the following day.

Failure to give adequate information to patients may result in claims for negligence if complications occur.

In addition to the mandatory written card, patients should be told how much load the cast will bear, how it should be supported for sleeping and protected from water.

Orthopedic department
Please read the following instructions carefully.
- Do not wet, cut, heat or otherwise interfere with this plaster.
- Report at once.
  - If it cracks, becomes loose or is otherwise uncomfortable.
  - If there is any pain.
  - If there is any discharge.
  - If the fingers or toes become numb or difficult to move.
  - If the fingers or toes become swollen or blue.
- The plaster may feel tight for some time after application.
- This can usually be relieved by lying down and elevating the arm or leg on one or more pillows and by constantly moving those joints of the arm and leg that are not covered by plaster.

Notice to patients wearing plaster casts
- For the first 24 hours keep the limb raised as much as possible keep the arm in the sling and the foot raised on a pillow or cushion protected with a waterproof cover. Keep the fingers and toes moving.
- If any of the following are noticed report condition to the emergency room or plaster room at once during day or night.
  - Swelling of the fingers or toes.
  - Blueness of the fingers or toes.
  - Pins and needles feeling in the fingers or toes.
  - Any real pain in the limb.
- Please visit the plaster room immediately next morning.

Patients with leg plasters will need crutches and demonstration of their use. Often, the physiotherapist will provide this service.

Complications
27. Name the complications of plasters.
Ans. Complications of plasters are as follows:

Venous Return

A moderate constriction will produce compression of the veins damming the blood, and causing swelling, discomfort or pain and a blue color in the skin under the nails.

Temporary remedies such as elevation of the limb and exercising the digits may be tried but if persistent the constriction must be relieved. The cast can be split and eased or bivalved taking care not to damage the skin.

Arterial Supply

A pale skin which is cool and pulseless indicates that the arterial supply is disrupted and following pressure on the finger nail the color does not immediately return. This is a serious complication. Medical advice must be sought immediately. Splitting the cast may be sought immediately. Splitting the cast may relieve the arterial compression, but surgery may be necessary sometimes. Incomplete arterial occlusion may present with pain or aching with loss of power. If in doubt, medical advice must be sought.

Pain

Pain may be due to tissue damage at injury or reduction, swelling within the cast, muscle spasm, pressure on blood vessels or nerves, skin irritation or sores. Although diagnosis may be difficult, persistent pain or intermittent acute pain should not be ignored.

Plaster Sores

The most common cause of sores is pressure of the plaster on the skin due to poor cast application. The patient may report burning, itching or stabbing pain. Children may have disturbed sleep and elevated temperature. Diagnosis is helped by looking for:
- Heat and swelling of the digits.
- Increased warmth over a localized area of the cast.
- Localized edema.
- Visible pus or staining of the cast.

The most likely reasons for plaster sore development are:

- *Poor technique* with inadequate padding or a ridge inside the cast, or failure to trim the ends of the cast correctly.
- *Inadequate instructions* to the patient may lead to local cast break down with skin irritation.
- *Inadequate supervision* by orthopedic staff such as failing to take corrective action at the first sign of skin irritation or cast loosening.
- *Foreign bodies* may easily slip between the cast and the skin. Children may insert small toys, coins or beads inside the cast. Patients should be warned of these damages and also to care for the plaster edges since wetting will cause plaster crumbs to be detached and fall inside the cast.
- *Scratching* at minor irritations beneath the cast with metal implements or knitting needles may cause trauma and infection. Such irritation should be reported and investigated early.
- *Cut edges* of plaster following splitting or bivalving or window procedures may irritate the skin especially if swelling occurs around the edge. If a window is not replaced the tissue is likely to become edematous and balloon through the window causing sores. The problem is accentuated in a load bearing plaster which may also be seriously weakened.

The patient is often able to pinpoint the sore area. The technician is usually asked to cut a window in the plaster. With an electric cutter a ten centimeter (4 inch) square can be removed intact. Then underlying padding and lining is removed to inspect the skin. After treatment the padding and window are replaced, secured by Elastoplast Elastic Adhesive Bandage or a circular turn of plaster bandage.

The alternative to cutting windows is to bivalve the cast enabling a full inspection. When the problem has been resolved a replacement cast will be necessary.

Loss of Position

Because swelling occurs with most fractures especially after reduction the technician puts padding under the cast to protect the skin. This padding gets compressed. After fortyeight hours when the edema is subsiding the cast may be too loose to hold the bone ends in position against undesirable muscle action. Such displacement may be sudden and cause pain or it may be gradual being first noticed on the check X-ray. This complication may seriously delay fracture union and may produce permanent deformity. Medical advice must be sought if the position is suspect.

Nerve Damage

Loss of power, tingling and numbness distal to the cast are signs of impaired nerve function. The cause may be direct compression by bone ends or plaster pressure, indirect compression of edematous tissue or tourniquet effect or reduced blood flow. Routine testing of power and sensation will detect any defect quickly. Corrective action includes relieving cast pressure, supporting and protecting paralyzed parts and physiotherapy to help restore normal function of muscle and joints.

Local Complications

Encasement of the limb or trunk in plaster may produce stiff joints, muscle wasting and impaired circulation. Physiotherapy and good nursing can help reduce these complications and speed the final recovery.

Systemic Complications

The most serious is deep venous thrombosis leading to pulmonary embolism. Pain in the calf is an important sign needing medical advice. Immobilization in trunk plasters or plasterbeds may also produce nausea, abdominal cramps, retention care of urine and abdominal distension. Good nursing, and diet with regular exercises will help ensure that the initial period of extensive immobilization is achieved without complications.

Removal of Plaster Casts

28. What are the methods of plaster removal?

Ans. All the equipment necessary for removing a cast should be close to hand. It should include scissors, benders, an electric cutter, materials for washing the limb and any supportive bandages or applications that may be necessary.

The limb in plaster should be supported by firm cushion. As most casts are removed by bivalving down the lateral sides, these areas should be easily accessible. The choice of apparatus depends on several factors. Casts can be cut with a plaster shear or an electric plaster cutter. While cutting a cast with an electric plaster cutter it must be ensured that the cast is sufficiently padded.

> **Note:** The noise of the electric plaster cutter frightens some patients and so shears may be used.

Explain the procedure to the patient and demonstrate the apparatus you will be using to make them feel at ease. Cut the cast steadily and smoothly and talk to the patient.

Use of Plaster Shears

29. Describe the use of plaster shears.

Ans. The size of shears used depends on the size of the cast. Draw guidelines down the side of the cast making sure that the line does not run directly over any bony prominences.

The stockinette is snipped at the ends of the cast to allow the shears to be positioned above this lining materials. If stockinette has not been used, try to insert the blade between the plaster and the undercast padding. Insert the blade under the plaster, parallel to the skin with the handle held steadily in the vertical position. The other blade cuts through the cast from above, its handle should be parallel to the skin at rest. This is the starting position and if the blades are incorrectly aligned the lower blade will press into the flesh causing bruises or even lacerations. After each cut, the blades should be realigned before the next cut is made. This prevents the skin wrinkling in front of the shears. These maneuvers are important because the thick tips of the shears can press uncomfortably on the surface of the skin. Remove the shears after every four or six cuts. Clear clogging in the blades and use the plaster blenders to open out the cast.

Never try to cut round corners. Always remove the blades and cut from the opposite end of the line to meet the end of the cut already made.

When using shears keep the elbow relatively still and apply the cutting force from the shoulder girdle and chest muscles. This gives a more controlled power and saves energy.

Use of the Electric Plaster Cutter
30. Describe the use of electric plaster cutter.

Ans. The electric cutter must only be used to cut completely padded casts.

Warning: If blood has impregnated the padding, it will be hard. Skin could adhere to it and the blades may cut directly into the skin.

When using an electric cutter make sure that.

- No strain is put on the cable and enough cable is available for comfortable use.
- The cable does not come near the cutting blade.
- Avoid usage in the presence of oxygen or inflammable gases.
- The operators hands are dry.
- The apparatus is serviced regularly.

Position the patient correctly, and mark the line of cutting. Reassure the patient by showing them that the cutting blade works by oscillation, and only cuts the materials. The blade becomes hot when used and cutting must be stopped if the patient feels any scorching. Start cutting with reduced pressure after examining the area involved. Position the blade at the start of the guideline, apply gentle pressure and move the cutter smoothly along the line. When cutting starts, there is a tendency to grip the cutter in a manner which exerts unwanted pressure on the cast. A new operator should be trained to reduce the pressure by continuous but gentle wrist movements.

The electric cutter should always be used carefully, especially near bony prominences such as the medial border of the foot leading to the big toe.

Care of the Part Replaced from the Cast

31. What is the after care following plaster removal?

Ans. The cast may have to be bivalved for inspection, X-ray purposes and some times for skin preparation prior to operation. In these circumstances, the halves are replaced and held by a bandage until further direction is given. On removal of the two parts of the cast, support the limb, between firm cushions and closely inspect it for any signs of trauma inflicted during the removal procedure. Wash and dry the part. Gently massage with oil, or a suitable lotion. This may help to restore normal nutrition and elasticity to the skin. After extended period of immobility, some edema is likely initially if the part is dependent.

Elastoplast

Elastic adhesive bandage or elastocrepe cotton bandage may be needed. These should support the whole area released from the cast. The new support should be applied at once and in the case of upper and lower limbs the patient should be advised to resume normal activity gradually, and to rest the part at regular intervals while maintaining digital exercises when at rest. When a plaster is removed before surgery, skin texture and nutrition should be improved by massage. This can help to stimulate good would healing after elective surgery.

Patients should always be warned that they may be incapacitated without the cast for the first few days until the muscles have regained their tone.

32. Mention the important rules of application of POP casts.

Ans. Following are the rules of application of POP casts:

Rules of application of POP casts
• Choose the correct size, 8 inches for the thigh, 6 inches for the leg, 4 inches for the forearm.
• A joint above and a joint below should be included.
• Accordingly, we have an above elbow or below elbow POP cast or slab and above knee or below knee POP cast or slab. This is done to eliminate movements of the joints on either side of the fractures. However, this is not a hard-and-fast rule in certain fractures, like a below elbow cast in Colles' fracture, which often suffices.
• It should be molded with the palm and not the fingers for fear of indentation.
• The joints should be immobilized in functional position.
• The plaster should just snugly fit and should not be too tight or too loose.
• Uniform thickness of the plaster is preferred.

Stage of Plastering

33. What are the stages of plaster application?

Ans. Stages of plaster application are as:

First Stage

The first stage involves application of POP slab or cast.

Second Stage or Cast-setting Stage

The second stage or cast-setting stage is change of POP to gypsum and is defined as the time taken to form rigid dressing after contact with water.

Third Stage or Green Stage
The third stage or green stage is the just set wet cast.

Fourth Stage or Cast Drying
The fourth stage or cast drying is by evaporation of excess of water when the cast dries. This results in a mature cast with multiple air pockets through which the skin breathes.

Complications of POP Casts

34. Name the complications of plaster of Paris casts.

Ans.

Due to tight fit
- Pain
- Pressure sores
- Compartmental syndromes
- Peripheral nerve injuries
- Cast syndrome

Due to improper application
- Joint stiffness
- Plaster blisters and sores
- Breakage

Due to plaster allergy
- Allergic dermatitis.

Remember

About POP
- Used first in city of Paris.
- The ideal splint.
- Slab for temporary and initial treatment.
- Casts for definitive treatment.
- Spica for hip fracture, etc.
- Functional cast brace for early mobilization.

FUNCTIONAL CAST BRACE

35. What are the principles of functional cast bracing?

Ans. If function is allowed during closed method of fracture treatment, it has been observed that, this stimulates osteogenesis, promotes soft tissue healing and prevents development of joint stiffness, loss of anatomic reduction to rapid healing. It complements rather than replacing other forms of treatment. The observation that fracture ribs still unite despite continuous movements, due to action of intercostal muscles, showed that elimination of movements at fracture site is not mandatory for a fracture to unite. It was on this brilliant concept that Sarmiento devised his unique functional bracing methods (Fig. 1.5).

MODE OF ACTION

36. What is the mode of action of functional cast brace?

Ans. Here the hydraulic action of muscles is brought into play. The fracture brace allows movements of the joints and permits the load to be transmitted through the muscles. The muscles which are surrounded by the inelastic deep fascia if encased in a hard plaster cannot be stretched beyond the confines of the cast. On movements and bearing weight, the

Remember

About functional cast brace

- Fracture ribs indicate that absolute immobility for fracture healing is not required.
- It is a secondary form of osteogenesis.
- Hydraulic action of muscles stabilizes the fracture in a closed compartment.
- Eliminates fracture disease.
- Not useful in compound fractures.
- Popularized by Sarmiento.
- Useful in fracture tibia and fracture femur.

muscle forces are hence driven inwards towards the fracture and not outwards. This helps the fracture to be held firmly. These hydraulic forces control the fragments and resist overlap and angulation till callus forms. Rotation is also resisted by the brace and muscle contraction.

> **Note:** In compound fractures due to severe disruption of soft tissues, this principle will not work until soft tissues have healed.

IMPORTANT SPLINTS IN ORTHOPEDICS OTHER THAN POP

THOMAS SPLINT

37. What is a Thomas splint?
Ans. Thomas splint is one of the very commonly used splints in orthopedics described by HO Thomas in 1876 to assist for ambulatory treatment of TB knee. It is now widely used for the treatment of shaft fractures of femur (Fig. 1.6).

Parts of Thomas Splint
38. What are the parts of a Thomas splint?
Ans. Thomas splint consists of four parts:
- A padded metal oval ring with soft leather set at an angle of 120° to the inner bar.
- The side bars—one inner and another outer bars of equal length. They bisect the oval ring.
- Distal end—where the two side bars are joined in the form of a "W".
- Outer side bar is angled 2 inches below the padded ring to clear the prominent greater trochanter.

Uses of Thomas Splint
39. Name the uses of a Thomas splint.
Ans. The uses of Thomas splint are:
- To immobilize fracture femur anywhere.
- As a first aid measure.

- For transportation of an injured patient.
- In the treatment of joint diseases like TB knee, etc.

BÖHLER-BRAUN (BB) SPLINT

40. What is a BB splint? Mention the use of the pulleys.
Ans. This is Böhler's modification of Braun splint. It consists of a heavy metallic frame with four pulleys:
- Proximal pulley prevents foot drop.
- Second pulley to apply traction in the line of femur.
- Third pulley to apply traction in the line of supracondylar area of femur.
- Fourth pulley to apply traction in line of the legs.
- Böhler-Braun splint is used to provide skeletal traction (*see* Fig. 2.6).

Indications
41. What are the indications of BB splint?
Ans. Skeletal traction is applied through this frame for comminuted trochanteric fractures of the femur. It is also used for the treatment of fracture shaft of femur and supracondylar fractures of the femur. Rarely, it can be used for the fracture shaft of tibia and fibula.

One important precaution which should be taken while using the BB splint is to provide support at the fracture site and not at the knee joint to prevent angulation, especially in supracondylar fractures of femur.

Problem of BB Splint
42. Name the problems with BB splint.
Ans. Following are the problems with BB splint.
- Makes nursing care difficult.
- It is a heavy and cumbersome frame.
- It is associated with recumbent problems like bed sores, hypostatic pneumonia, renal calculi, etc.
- It can cause stiffness of the knee.

Care of the Splints

43. Mention the care of BB splints.

Ans.

- *Padding:* The splint should be well padded at the bony prominences and at the injury sites.
- *Bandage:* This should be tied with optimum pressure.
- *Exercises:* Active exercises of the joints and muscles should be permitted within the splints.
- *Checking:* Daily checking and adjustments of the splints are recommended.
- *Neurovascular status:* Distal neurovascular status should be assessed daily.

OTHER SPLINTS

44. Name the other common splints used in orthopedics and their indication.

Ans. Other common splints used in orthopedics are:

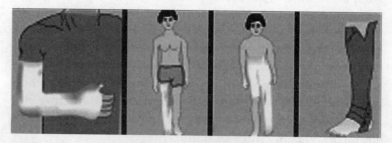

Fig. 1.1: Types of plaster casts

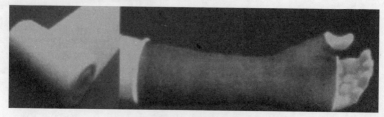

Fig. 1.2: Fiberglass plasters

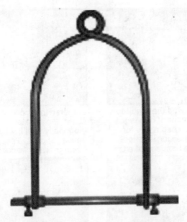

Fig. 1.3: Böhler's stirrup and Denham pin

Region	Indications
Cervical spine	
• SOMI brace	Cervical spine injury
• 4 post collar	Neck immobilization
Upper limbs	
• Aeroplane splint	Brachial plexus injury
• Cock-up splint	Radial nerve palsy
• Kunckle-bender splint	Ulnar nerve palsy
• Aluminium splint	Finger injury
• Volkmann's splint	For VIC
Spine	
• Milwaukes brace	Scoliosis
• Boston brace	Scoliosis
• Taylor brace	Dorsolumbar injury
• Anterior spinal hyperextension brace (ASHE)	Dorsolumbar injury
• Lumbar belts and corsets	Backache
Lower limb	
• Trochanteric	BB splint fracture
• Foot drop splint	Foot drop
Miscellaneous	
• Thomas splint	For lower limb injuries
• Krammer wire splint	For emergencies as a first aid measure

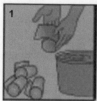

Unwrap the required number of bandages and keep ready for immersion. Wet only one bandage at a time

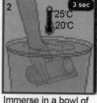

Immerse in a bowl of clean, tepid water diagonally until bubbles cease (approx. 3 sec). Change water frequently

Remove bandage and gently squeeze it from edges to centre to expel surplus water.

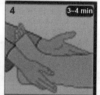

Normal setting time is 3–4 minutes. To retard, use common borax

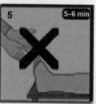

Do not mould the cast after 5–6 minutes

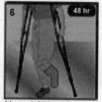

No weight bearing before 48 hours

Fig. 1.4: Stages of plastering

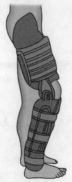

Fig. 1.5: Functional cast brace

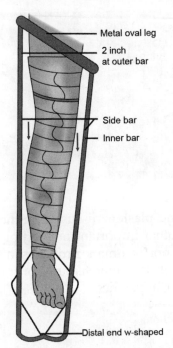

Fig. 1.6: Thomas splint

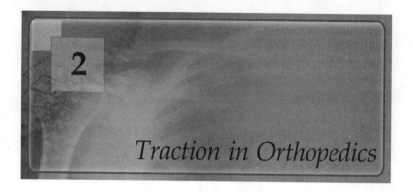

2

Traction in Orthopedics

Like splints and plasters discussed in the previous chapter traction is another important method of treatment of both traumatic and non traumatic problems in orthopaedics. This chapter highlights various features of traction as a form of treatment in orthopaedics

Methods of Traction
- Skin tractions
- Skeletal traction

Let us begin with the most likely questions that will be asked in viva voce.

1. What is traction?
Traction is a method of applying sustaned force to a part of the body with an external device.
Ans. Traction plays an important role in the management of fractures in orthopedics.
Use of traction

2. What are the uses of traction?
Ans. Following are the uses of traction:
- To reduce a fracture or a dislocation.
- To retain the fracture after reduction.
- To overcome the muscle spasm.
- To control movement of an injured part of the body and to aid in healing.

METHODS OF TRACTION

3. Name the methods of traction.

Ans. There are four methods of applying traction, namely skin, skeletal, pelvic and spinal.

SKIN TRACTION

4. What is skin traction?

Ans. Here traction is applied over a large area of skin. Maximum weight that can be applied through skin traction is 15 lb or 6.7 kg. If the weight used is more than this, the traction will slide down peeling off the skin. When used in fracture, skin traction is applied to the limb distal to the fracture site.

Types of Skin Traction

5. Name the types of skin traction.

Ans. There are two types of skin traction.

Adhesive Skin Traction

Here adhesive material is used for strapping which is applied anteromedial and posterolateral on either side of the lower limb.

Nonadhesive Skin Traction

Useful in thin and atrophic skin and in patients sensitive to adhesive strap. It is less secure than the former.

Contraindications for Skin Traction

6. Mentions the contraindication for skin traction.

Ans. Abrasions, lacerations, impaired circulation, infection dermatitis, marked shortening, allergy to plaster are some of the important contraindications for skin traction.

Complications

7. Name the complications of skin traction.

Ans. Allergy, excoriations, pressure sores around the malleoli, common peroneal nerve palsy, etc. are some of the known complications in skin traction.

> **Remember**
> • Rotation of the limb is difficult to control with skin tractions.

Important Skin Tractions

8. Name the important skin tractions.

Ans. Some of the important skin tractions are given below:

Buck's Extension Skin Traction

Bucks extension skin traction is the commonest type of traction employed for lower limbs. It is used for temporary treatment of fracture neck femur, undisplaced fractures of acetabulum, after reduction of hip dislocation, to correct minor fixed flexion deformity of hip and knee for low backache, etc (Fig. 2.1).

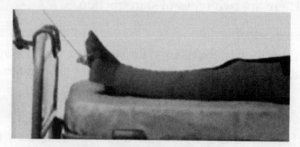

Fig. 2.1: Buck's skin traction

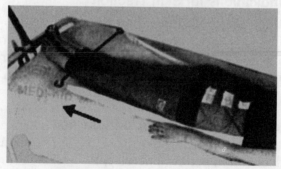

Fig. 2.2: Lumbar or pelvic traction

Dunlop's Traction

Used in upper limbs and is indicated for supracondylar fractures, intercondylar fractures of humerus where elbow flexion causes circulatory embarrassment (Fig. 2.3).

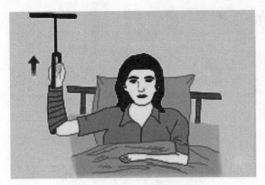

Fig. 2.3: Dunlop's traction

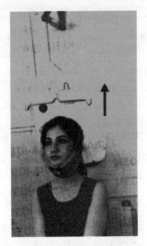

Fig. 2.4: Cervical traction

Gallow's Traction of Bryant's Traction

Used for fracture of shaft femur in children less than 2 years. If used in children above 2 years, it causes vascular complications (Fig. 2.5).

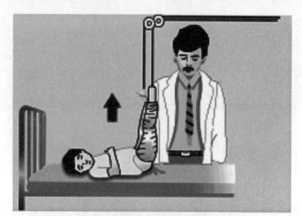

Fig. 2.5: Gallow's traction

SKELETAL TRACTION

9. What is skeletal traction?

Ans. Here the traction is given through a metal or pin driven through the bone. It is seldom necessary for upper limb fractures but useful in lower limb fractures for reducing and maintaining the fracture reduction. It is reserved for those cases in which skin traction is contraindicated and where the need to be applied weight is more than 5 kg.

Know the Pins Used for Skeletal Traction

10. What are the pins used for skeletal traction?

Ans. Following pins are used for applying skeletal traction:

Steinmann Pin

Steinmann pin is a rigid stainless steel pin 4 to 6 mm in diameter. Böhler's stirrup allows the direction of the traction to be varied without turning the pin in the bone (*see* Fig. 1.3).

Denham Pin

Denham pin is threaded in the center and engages the bony cortex. It reduces the risk of pin sliding and is useful in cancellous bone like calcaneum and osteoporotic bones.

K-wire

K-wire is of small diameter and is often used in upper limbs.

TRACTION POINTS WELL KNOWN IN ORTHOPEDICS

11. Name the important skeletal traction in orthopedics.
Ans. Following skeletal traction are important in orthopedics:

Tractions	Indications
Head and cervical tractions	
• Crutchfield or Gardenwells	Cervical spine injury
• Head halter	Cervical spine injury
• Halopelvic	Scoliosis
Upper limb tractions	
• Olecranom traction	Supracondylar fracture
• Metacarpal traction	Compound forearm injuries
Lower limb tractions	
• Trochanteric traction	Central dislocation hip
• Supracondylar traction	Trocharteric/femur fractures
• Upper tibial traction	Trochartoric and femur fractures
• Lower tibial traction	Froximal tibial fractures
• Calcaneal traction	Compound fractures of distal leg and ankle
• Metatarsal tractions	For distal tibial and heel injuries.

Know the Sites and Indications for Skeletal Traction

12. Mention the important sites and indications for skeletal traction.
Ans.

Sites of skeletal traction	Exact point and indication
Skull traction	
Outer table of parietal bone of the skull	To reduce dislocation with either Crutchfield for Gardenwells tongs of cervical spine
	• For postoperative treatment
	• For cervical spondylosis with severe nerve root compression

Upper limbs	
• Olecranon	1¼" distal to the tip of olecranon, Supracondylar, intercondylar and comminuted fracture lower third of humerus
• Second and third metacarpals	1" proximal to the distal end of forearm, fracture both bones forearm, second metacarpals

Lower limbs	
• Greater trochanter	1" below the most prominent part of the greater trochanter, midway between anterior and posterior surfaces of femur. Central fracture dislocation of hip
• Lower end of femur	1" above the knee joint pelvic fractures, posterior dislocation of hip, trochanteric fractures, shaft fractures, etc.
• Upper end of tibia	¾" below and lateral to the tibial tuberosity. All of the above indications, supracondylar fractures and intercondylar fractures of the femur
• Lower end of tibia	2" above the level of ankle joint mid-way between anterior and posterior border
	Tibial plateau fractures Fracture both bones leg
• Calcaneum	2 cm below and behind the lateral malleolus fracture lower one-third of the leg and ankle injuries
• Metatarsal bones	Through the base of the metatarsals for calcaneal fractures

Note: Commonest site for skeletal traction is upper end of tibia and the common indication for skeletal traction is trochanteric fractures in elderly persons.

13. Mention in brief the steps of upper tibial skeletal traction.

Ans.

- Patient is in major or minor OT.
- The part is shared, painted and draped.
- Local anesthetic is injected at the point of insertion.
- A small nick is made with a scalpel about 1.5 cm below and lateral to the tibial tubercle.

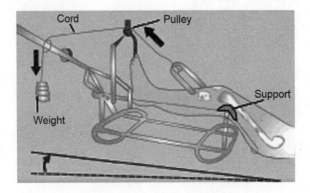

Fig. 2.6: Skeletal traction on Böhler-Braun frame

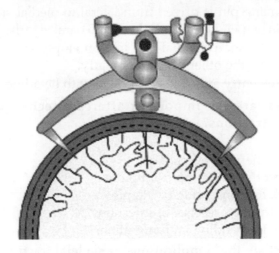

Fig. 2.7: Crutchfield tongs

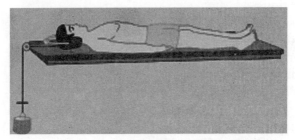

Fig. 2.8: Application of Crutchfield tongs

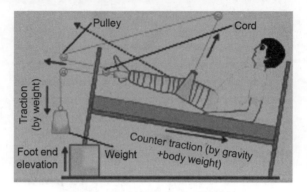

Fig. 2.9: Balanced traction

- Steinmann pin is driven from lateral to medial side with the pin perpendicular to the bone and parallel to the ground.
- Insert the sharp medial end into an empty injection vial to protect the other limb from injury.
- Seal the entry and exit skin points with betadine seal.

14. What are the important aftercare techniques for skeletal tractions?

Ans.

- Check the pins everyday.
- Inspect the entry and exit points.
- Check for conserving of the pins.
- Look for the presence of infections.
- Check for bending and migration.

15. What are the complications of skeletal tractions?

Ans.

- Infections
- Loosening
- Bending
- Migration
- Breakage
- Epiphyseal injury in children
- Injury to the lateral popliteal nerve
- Injury to the vessels
- Injury to the unaffected leg

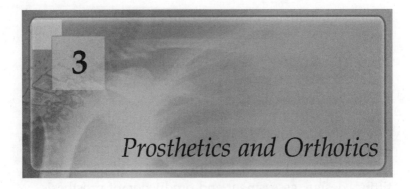

3

Prosthetics and Orthotics

This chapter deals with prosthetics and orthotics which place a very important role in the treatment of various neuromuscular and situations of limb loss in orthopedics. This book gives an insight into the various aspects of the prosthetics and orthotics.

Prosthetics

- Classification
- Types
- Prosthesis for the lower limbs
- Prosthesis for disarticulation of hip and hemipelvectomy
- Above knee transfemoral amputation
- Prosthesis for Syme's amputation
- Prosthesis for partial foot amputation
- Prosthesis for bilateral amputation
- Prosthesis for upper limb amputation
- Re-education of patients
- Re-educating an upper limb amputee

Orthotics

- Classification
- Terminology for orthosis
- Qick facts
- Action of orthosis
- Spinal orthosis
- Orthosis for cervical spine

Footwear and its Modifications

- Braces

Let us begin with the most likely questions that will be asked in viva voce.

PROSTHETICS

1. What is prosthesis? Define it.
Ans. Prosthesis in Greek means "in addition". Thus prosthesis is defined as a replacement or substitution of a missing or a diseased part.

Prosthesis is the theory and practice of the prescription, fitting, design, assessment and production of prosthesis.

Classification
2. What are the types of prosthesis?
Ans. There are two types of prosthesis.

Endoprosthesis

Endoprosthesis is implants used in orthopedic surgery to replace joints, e.g. Austin-Moore prosthesis.

Exoprosthesis

Exoprosthesis is for replacement externally for a lost part of the limb. They are more extensively used in the lower limbs.

3. Name the different materials used for making prosthesis.
Ans. Different materials used for making prosthesis are:

Wood
• Socket material
• Prosthetic foot

Leather
• Soft variety—suspension straps
• Hard variety—thigh and socket corsets

Plastic
• Plastic foam—for support of the distal stump
• Polypropylene—for making of sockets

Metal
- Steel—for knee and hip mechanism
- Duraluminium—for outer shelf and socket

4. What are the factors considered before fitting a prosthesis?

Ans. Following factors are considered before a prosthetic fitting.
- Age of the patient
- Sex
- General build
- Personal and professional requirement of the patient
- Circulation status of the stump
- Range of motion (ROM) of all the joints and the affected limb.
- The muscle strength of the affected limb.

> *Note*
> Suction socket is not indicated for ischemic limbs.

Types

Temporary Prosthesis

5. What is a temporary prosthesis?

Ans. Temporary prosthesis, e.g. pylon, is used following an amputation, till the patient is fitted with permanent prosthesis after 2 weeks of removal of the suture (Fig. 3.1).

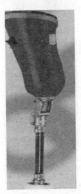

Fig. 3.1: Temporary prosthesis

Permanent Prosthesis

6. What is a permanent prosthesis?

Ans. Permanent prosthesis is fitted after making a final clinical assessment.

PROSTHESIS FOR LOWER LIMBS

7. Name the different prostheses for the lower limbs.
Ans.
- Prosthesis for hip disarticulation and semi pelvectomy
- Above knee transfemoral prosthesis
- Below knee prosthesis
- Syne's prosthesis

PROSTHESIS FOR DISARTICULATION OF HIP AND HEMIPELVECTOMY (Fig. 3.2)

8. Describe the prostheses for disarticulation of hip and hemipelvectomy

Ans. These prostheses should have the following designs.

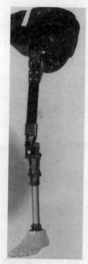

Fig. 3.2: Prosthesis for hemipelvectomy and hip disarticulation

Socket

- Totally embracing socket enclosing both iliac crests.
- Weight-bearing areas:
  - Hemipelvectomy: Ischial tuberosity and buttock of the other side.
  - Hip disarticulation: Ischium and buttock of the same side.

Suspension

- Suspension is through the total tissue contact with locking on the iliac crests.

Hip Joint

Two types of locking are in use:
- *Standard locking*: This locks automatically on hip extension.
- *Canadian locking*: This also locks automatically when the patient stands and is placed anteriorly. During swing phase of the gait, it allows 20° of flexion.

Knee Joint

To offer stability during the stance phase, the knee joint is placed in hyperextension. This lock could be manual, semiautomatic or automatic.

Feet

To offer maximum stability during standing, solid ankle cushion heel (SACH) is preferred.

Note
- Uniaxial foot—permits only dorsiflexion and plantar flexion.
- Biaxial foot—permits the above and also foot inversion and eversion.
- Double swivel joint—permits all movements of the hip.
- Rigid pelvic band—permits only hip flexion and extension.

ABOVE KNEE TRANSFEMORAL AMPUTATION (Fig. 3.3)

9. Describe the prosthesis for above knee transfemoral amputation.

Ans. The following two types of prostheses are recommended.

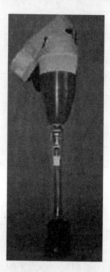

Fig. 3.3: Above knee prosthesis

Suction-socketed Limb

Suction-socketed limb is useful in young adults and is best suited for cylindrical stumps. It snugly fits and has a two-way valve mechanism to maintain negative pressure.

Non-suction Limb

Here no negative pressure is employed to hold the prosthesis, but pelvic band or harness are made use of for holding.

The advantages of suction-socketed limb are that skin infection is less common, there is freedom from harness of any kind, greater feel of close contact of the prosthesis and the patient feels that it belongs to him or her. Stump socks are not necessary in this variety. On the contrary, the advantages of non-suction-socketed limb are it is easy to wear, there is no perspiration, it provides a comfortable fit, and there is no difficulty in changing the stump circumference.

Components of Prosthesis

10. Name the components of prosthesis.

Ans. Components of a prosthesis are:

- *Socket*: This provides a receptive area for the stump and helps in weight bearing.
- *Suspension*: This fastens the prosthesis to the stump.
- *Joints*: These are artificial mechanical joints which replace the original joints.
- *Base*: This is in touch with the floor.

Note: **Types of artificial joints**

- Manually operated.
- Semiautomatic.
- Automatic.

11. Compare the prosthesis for knee disarticulation and above knee amputation.

Ans.

Table 3.1

Features	Knee disarticulation	A/K amputation
Socket	Thigh corset H socket	Quadrilateral
Suspension	Rigid pelvic band or shoulder suspension or waist band	Double swivel pelvic band Suction socket valve
Knee	Unilateral joint with manual or automatic locking	Modular prosthesis Hand operated or semiautomatic locking
Feet	SACH foot or uniaxial foot	SACH or uniaxial foot

Prosthesis for Through Knee

12. Mention about the prosthesis for through knee amputation.

Ans. As already mentioned, knee disarticulation gives a good, stable, long weight-bearing stump which enables to operate the prosthesis with comfort.

Prosthesis for Below Knee Amputation (Figs 3.5 to 3.7)

13a. Mention the types of below knee prosthesis.

Ans. Two varieties are described here.

Patellar Tendon Bearing Prosthesis

In patellar tendon bearing (PTB) prosthesis, the socket is made in such a way that it fits exactly over the patellar tendon and the sides of the tibial condyles, such that when in full extension the weight is transferred to some extent through this to the prosthesis. This has the advantage over the conventional prosthesis which require the knee supports (Fig. 3.4).

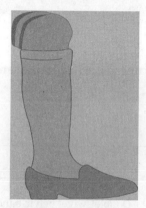

Fig. 3.4: PTB prosthesis

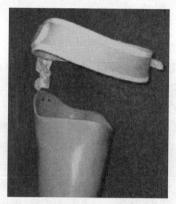

Fig. 3.5: Nonsuction below knee prosthesis

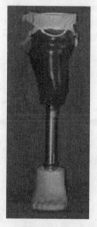

Fig. 3.6: Below knee prosthesis

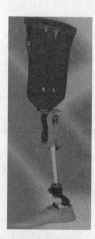

Fig. 3.7: Prosthesis for below knee amputation

Conventional Type Prosthesis

Conventional type prosthesis consists of the thigh corset, the side steels, the knee joint, shin piece, ankle joint unit and the foot piece. It definitely has the disadvantage in that it is more cumbersome to put on and use it when compared to the PTB prosthesis (Fig. 3.5)

13b. Compare conventional and PTB prosthesis
Ans.

Table 3.2

Features	Conventional prosthesis	PTB prosthesis
Socket	Extends 3 cm above the lower pole of patella A metal, wood and polyester proximal weight-bearing socket	Soft inner socket with a hard covering
Suspension	Rigid pelvic band if required, shoulder strap or waist belt	Elastic stocking Suspension and supracondylar cuff
Knee	Uniaxial joint	—
Feet	Uniaxial foot	Uniaxial Multiaxial SACH foot

PROSTHESIS FOR SYME'S AMPUTATION

14. What is Syme's prosthesis?

Ans. This is a below knee prosthesis used after Syme's amputation. This prosthesis has closed sockets or open sockets and may be full weight bearing or modified end bearing (Fig. 3.8)

Quick facts

- Quadrilateral socket prosthesis for above knee amputation.
- PTB prosthesis for below knee amputation.
- Syme's prosthesis for Syme's amputation.
- Shoe fillers for partial foot amputation.

Indications for conventional prosthesis

- Heavy manual labourers.
- Patellar defects.
- FFD of knee >25°
- Unstable knee
- Very short stump
- Anesthetic stump

Advantages of PTB prosthesis

- Permits normal gait.
- Permits early rehabilitation.
- Convenient for patients with a long stump.

Quick facts

Prosthesis for Syme's amputation

- *Enclosed metal Syme:* In this there is a leather liner with a posterior flap. Uniaxial foot is used.
- *Tongue and butt Syme:* Here two side steels connect the socket to the foot piece. It has a leather socket which opens in front.
- *Plastic Syme:* There is a hard plastic outer socket with a thin pelite liner inside with medial or posterior access panel.
- *Three strip posterior steel socket:* This is connected in front by two die steels and an inverted Y-shaped front steel parts.
  The socket which is made up of leather has an opening posteriorly and is fully articulated to the foot.

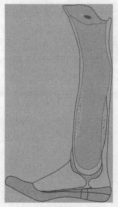

Fig. 3.8: Syme's prosthesis

PROSTHESIS FOR PARTIAL FOOT AMPUTATION

15. Name the prosthesis for partial foot amputation.

Ans. Two varieties are described: Shoe fillers made up of leather. Ankle corset attached to the wooden foot inside the foot.

PROSTHESIS FOR BILATERAL AMPUTATIONS

16. Name the types of prosthesis for bilateral amputations.
Ans.

For Bilateral above Knee Amputations

- Wheelchair for elderly patients.
- Short arm crutches with plastozoate stump covers.

For Bilateral Hip Amputations

- Axillary crutches.
- Ambulation through a fiberglass special sitting shell and push up blocks.

Ankle Units and Artificial Feet

17. What is SACH foot?

Ans. Solid action cushion heel (SACH) foot has no ankle joint but a simulated action is gained by the compression of wedge-shaped rubber heel and the whole foot is incorporated with various layers of rubber with its density varying, all placed over a wooden insert for the heel and wooden insert for the heel and wooden side keel. This allows smooth movements of the foot (Figs 3.9 and 3.10)

Remember

Aims of prosthetic fitting
- To substitute for a lost part.
- To restore a lost function.
- In lower limbs it must provide a comfortable ambulation with minimal expenditure of energy

In prosthesis for lower extremities.
Long stump is prosthetically superior to a shorter one because it provides.
- Longer lever arm.
- More sensory feedback.
- Greater area for distribution of pressure forces.

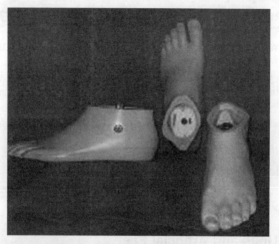

Fig. 3.9: SACH foot, Seattle foot and carbon foot

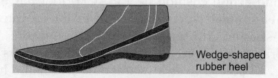

Wedge-shaped rubber heel

Fig. 3.10: SACH foot

JAIPUR FOOT (Fig. 3.11)

- This is the brainchild of Dr PK Sethi and Masterji Ram Chander Sharma of Jaipur.
- Rubber and aluminum is the mainstay. Rubber is waterproof; aluminum is used for the leg piece, because it is cheap, strong and rustproof.

- Unlike the western model, Jaipur foot is best for foot conditions in developing countries as it allows sitting on the floor, squatting and does not require a shoe.

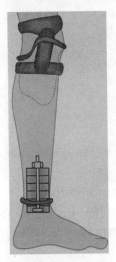

Fig. 3.11: Jaipur foot

PROSTHESIS FOR UPPER LIMB AMPUTATIONS

18. Name the prosthesis used for upper limbs.

Ans. Following prostheses are used for upper limbs.

For Forequarter Amputations

Here the prosthesis merely serves a cosmetic purpose. A sleeve fitter prosthesis with a plastozoate cap padded inside with foam and retaining straps is used.

For Shoulder Disarticulation (Fig. 3.12)

- Shoulder piece—extended cap to hold the prosthesis.
- Elbow piece—can be flexed by pulling on the flexion cord with the protractors of the shoulder.
- Hand piece—either cosmetic or splint hook type.

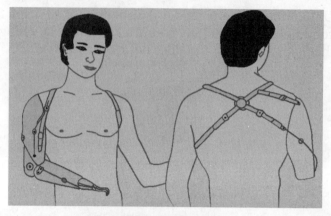

Fig. 3.12: Above elbow prosthesis

For Above Elbow Amputation

Same as above except that the elbow flexion is stronger due to the action of the arm muscles along with the protractors of the shoulder.

For Below Elbow Amputation

- Here there is a cup socket attached to the terminal device through an operational cord.
- The terminal device can be activated through a loop harness.

For Wrist Disarticulation

In this, a split socket forearm and a wrist rotation device is provided. A device can be provided to lock for supination and pronation.

Re-education of Patients

19. What does a patient wearing the prosthesis need to learn?
Ans.
- How to apply and remove the prosthesis correctly.
- How to identify complications arising out of fitting and use of prosthesis.

- How to walk over with the prosthesis.
- How to maintain and take care of the prosthesis.
- To acquire functional training in upper limb amputees.
- A knowledge about the structure and function of the prosthesis.

Quick facts

The terminal devices for the upper limb prosthesis:

- Splint hook: This has two jaws, one is fixed and the other one moves by the power of shoulder girdle muscles. This is a popular device.
- Mechanical thumb abduction device.
- Mechanical hand providing flexion of the thumb, middle and index fingers.
- A battery operated myoelectric device for grip.

Vital points before prosthetic application:

- Check the joint alignment and its movements.
- The socks should be pulled up and fastened firmly.
- The prosthesis is applied in the functional position.
- Upper limb prosthesis applied in sitting position.
- Lower limb prosthesis applied in standing with 2″ apart in parallel bars.
- Check the anatomical alignment in respect to normal limbs.
- Check the heels of the body from front, back, sides.
- Check for any discomfort in weight bearing areas.
- Check the axis for weight bearing and prosthetic joint.
- Check the overall fitting of the socket.
- Check for the proper fitting for the corset.
- Check for the proper fitting of the suspension.
- Check the prosthetic joints.
- Check the length of the prosthesis especially that of the lower limbs.
- Check the SACH, uniaxial or biaxial foot.

---

20. How is a patient trained to walk on a prosthesis?

Ans. A patient is trained to walk on a prosthesis as follows:

- Training is given in the parallel bars.
- First, standing balance on both the legs is taught.
- Second, taking the body weights on both the legs alternatively.

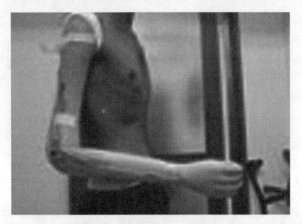

Fig. 3.13: Below elbow prosthesis

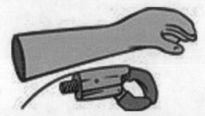

Fig. 3.14: Motorised hand

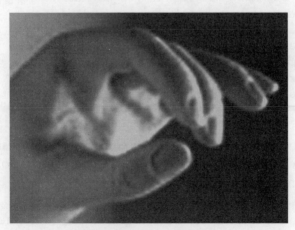

Fig. 3.15: Prosthetic hand

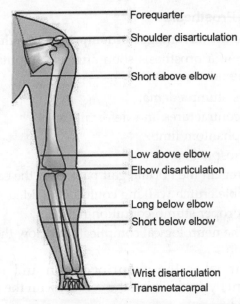

Fig. 3.16: Levels of amputation of upper limb

- Third, with bilateral hand support, coordinated stepping is taught.
- Fourth, it is now progressed to single hand support.
- Fifth, sitting to standing and vice versa is taught.
- Sixth, turning, side walking, climbing taught next.
- Once the patient has gained sufficient mastery in the parallel bars, he is next made to walk on the foot-marks over the floor in front of a mirror.
- PNF techniques of resistive gait is practised.

The physiotherapist should be able to identify if there is any gait deviation from the normal gait pattern, detect the cause for it and rectify it.

Note
Patient is taught balance and equilibrium during all the above activities.

Temporary Prosthesis

21. What are the advantages of temporary prosthesis?

Ans. Fitting of a prosthesis soon after an amputation has the following advantages.

- Minimizes stump edema.
- Prevents contractures and deformities.
- Prevents phantom limb.
- Reduces hospital stay.
- Helps to regain the normal gait pattern at the earliest.
- The unstable crutch walking could be avoided.
- Helps in proper stump conditioning.
- Reduces the neurological complication below the level of amputation.
- It re-establishes the proprioception and feedback mechanism by establishing the contact with the proximal part quickly.
- It helps in ambulation, weight transfer and stabilization.

22. How to construct a temporary prosthesis?

Ans. A good temporary prosthesis is constructed as follows:

- A good functional stump is first created.
- A sterile stump sock is applied.
- A rigid dressing is done by applying a POP cast.
- Into the above cast is incorporated a device with steel straps.
- To this is applied a pre-measured walking plaster with SACH foot.
- After three weeks, the cast is split and measurements are taken for the final prosthesis.

> *Note*
>
> **On temporary prosthesis.**
> - Standing and partial weight bearing is begun the next day.
> - Full weight bearing by six weeks.

Re-educating an Upper Limb Amputee

23. What is the goal of re-educating a upper limb amputee.

Ans. Here the goal is to train the patient for functional activities.

24. What are the principles of upper limb amputations?

Ans. The above goal can be achieved by observing the following principles:

- For the absence of the true limb, the adjacent parts should be trained to increase their mobility.
- Strengthening exercises to the muscles needed for operating the prosthesis.
- To prevent contractures in the important muscle groups like shoulder adductors, elbow flexors, etc.

For Above Elbow Amputation

25. What is the rehabilitation program for above elbow amputation?

Ans. Here, the movements of the neck, trunk, scapulohumeral and scapulothoracic muscles should be strengthened.

The flexors, extensors and adductors of the shoulder are put through vigorous muscle strengthening and endurance exercises to bring about flexion of the prosthesis at the elbow.

For Below Elbow Amputation

26. What is the rehabilitation program for below elbow amputation? How do you teach a patient to operate an upper limb prosthesis?

Ans. Here, along with the above, strengthening exercises are given for the elbow flexors, extensors and forearm muscles.

Teaching a patient how to operate the prosthesis of the upper limb consists of the below steps:

- First step, train the patient how to perform true shoulder flexion (i.e. without movement at the shoulder girdle).

- Second, the patient with below elbow amputation, training is given to flex the elbow to 90° and then flex the shoulder to activate the terminal device.
- Third, in patients with above elbow amputation, by following the first step mentioned above, patient is taught to flex the elbow of the prosthesis.
- Then, with the prosthetic elbow locked, the terminal device is activated by flexion at the shoulder.
- This is the dual control system.
- Triple control system for the above elbow amputee:
  - Flex the elbow by true shoulder flexion.
  - Lock the prosthetic elbow by arm extension control motion.
  - Activate the terminal device by shrugging the normal shoulder.

ORTHOTICS

27. Define an orthosis.
Ans. Orthosis is an appliance which is added to the patient to enable better use of that part of the body to which it is fitted.

- Prosthesis replaces a missing part of the body.
- An orthotist is a person qualified to measure and fit all types of orthoses.

Classification
28. Name the classifications for orthosis.
Ans. One single classification is very difficult. Hence, GK Rose has grouped them as follows:

- Functional biomechanical.
- Functional descriptive.
- Nosological (according to disease)
- Regional

Terminology for Orthosis

29. What are the terminologies used for orthosis?

Ans. The three major anatomical regions of the body are divided as follows and the initials given are as below:

Table 3.3: Orthotic terminologies

Upper limbs	Lower limbs	Spine
S—shoulder	H—hip	C—cervical
E—elbow	K—knee	T—thoracic
W—wrist	A—ankle	L—lumbar
H—hand	F—foot	S—sacroiliac
F—fingers MP	Subtalar	
(2–5) DIP	Midtarsal	
PIP	Metatarsal	
Thumb CM		
MP		
IP		

Action of Orthosis

30. Name the action of an orthosis.

Ans. Action of an orthosis on a joint is indicated by initials which are as follows:

- F—free
- A—Assist
- R—Resist
- S—Stop
- H—Hold
- V—Variable
- L—Lock

Quick facts

Nomenclature for orthosis now used has the first letter of the name of each joint which the orthosis crosses in power sequence, and the letter 'O' for orthosis is attached at the end. Accordingly, we have the following types of orthoses:

- CO—cervical orthosis.
- CTLSO—cervico-thoraco-lumbar-sacral orthoses.
- WHO—wrist-hand orthoses.

- HKAFO—hip-knee-ankle-foot orthoses.
- KAFO—knee-ankle-foot orthoses.
- KO—knee orthosis.
- AFO—ankle-foot orthoses.

SPINAL ORTHOSES

31. Name the spinal orthoses
Ans. Spinal orthoses fall into two categories:
- Supportive
- Corrective

Functions of Spinal Orthosis

32. What are the functions of spinal orthosis?
Ans. The functions of spinal orthosis are as follows
- To relieve pain
- To support weakened paralyzed muscles
- To support unstable joints
- To immobilize joints in functional position
- To prevent deformity
- To correct deformity

Supportive Spinal Orthosis

33. Name the supportive spinal orthosis?
Ans. *Belts and corsets:* Belts and corsets are most commonly used for the treatment of low backache. Belts are prescribed for men and corsets for women. These orthoses encircle the sacral region and extend a variable distance upwards, the term applied to them depends upon their depth posteriorly (sacroiliac, lumbosacral, thoracolumbar). Anteriorly, they have buckles.

Remember
The role of belts
• They do not immobilize the spine but only restrict extremes of forward, lateral flexion and extension.
• They supply subjective support.
• They remind the patients to avoid movements.

Rigid Spinal Brace

All rigid spinal orthoses are constructed on the basis of a metal frame which takes firm support from the pelvis. To this is added the metal uprights which are joined by cross bars and straps, e.g. tailor brace, night tailor brace.

Moulded Spinal Orthosis

Moulded spinal orthosis are made of leather, plastics, etc. and can be moulded to part of the body.

34. What are the indications for supportive spinal orthosis.

Ans. Indications for supportive spinal orthosis are:

- Sacroiliac strain.
- Low backache.
- Prolapsed intervertebral disc.
- Spondylolisthesis, etc.

Remember

The mechanisms of pain relief by spportive spinal orthoses.

- Psychological.
- Increases intraabdominal pressure.
- Decreases lumbar lordosis.
- Causes local inactivity of associated muscle groups and ligaments.

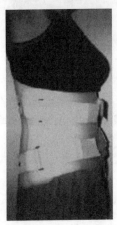

Fig. 3.17a: Lumbosacral orthosis custom made plastic

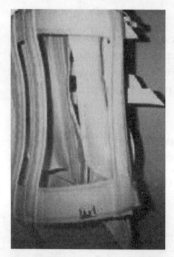

Fig. 3.17b: Chairback brace

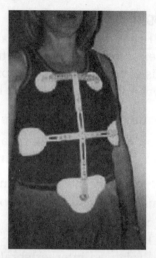

Fig. 3.17c: Cruciform anterior hyperextension brace

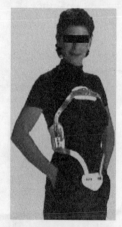

Fig. 3.18: Jewett hyper-extension brace

Corrective Spinal Orthosis

35. What is a Milwaukee brace?

Ans. Milwaukee brace is an active corrective spinal orthosis used almost exclusively in the ambulant treatment of structural scoliosis (Fig. 3.19).

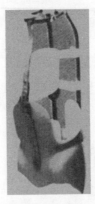

Fig. 3.19: Milwaukee brace

The main aim of Milwaukee brace is to postpone, temporarily or permanently, the need for an operation.

VARIOUS TYPES OF SPINE ORTHOSIS

ORTHOSIS FOR CERVICAL SPINE

36. Name the orthosis for cervical spine

Ans. Orthosis for cervical spine are (Fig. 3.27)

- *Cervical collar:* Many different forms of cervical collars or supports are available and are called Thomas collars. Metal was used earlier, but now thick plastic sheets are preferred. These collars are ready-made and are supplied in different sizes or are adjustable. For a good fit, the collar should be secured firmly around the neck, rest upon the chest and shoulders and support the chin, jaw and occiput.
- SOMI (sterno-occiput mandibular immobilization) brace (Fig. 3.20).
- Four postcervical brace (Fig. 3.21).
- Halo body orthosis Fig. 3.24).
- *Minerva jacket:* In lesions of uppermost part of the cervical spine, the forehead must be included in the external support. In such situations, Minerva jacket made from plaster of Paris is used (Fig. 3.25).

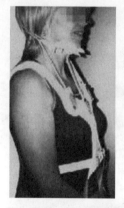

Fig. 3.20: Somi brace

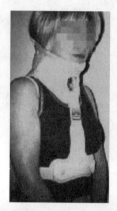

Fig. 3.21: Philadelphia collar

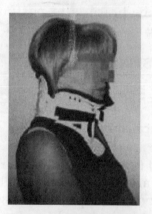

Fig. 3.22: Miami collar

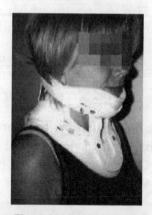

Fig. 3.23: Malibu collar

LOWER LIMB ORTHOSIS

37. What is a caliper?
Ans. Caliper is an orthosis for the lower limb which may be used permanently or for a very short time only.

38. What are the functions of a caliper?
Ans. The functions of a caliper are:
- It provides stability.
- It relieves weight bearing.

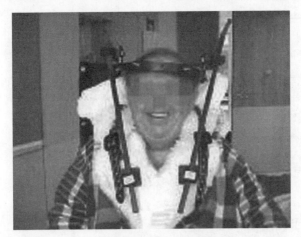

Fig. 3.24: Halo device

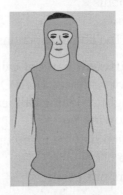

Fig. 3.25: Minerva jacket

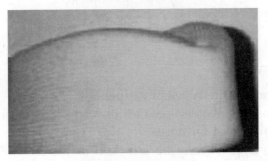

Fig. 3.26: Soft collar

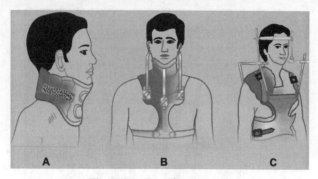

Fig. 3.27: Cervical orthosis

- It relieves pain.
- It controls deformity.
- It restricts movements.
- It assists movements.
- A combination of the above functions.

39a. What are the different parts of caliper?

Ans. Knee-ankle-foot orthoses (KAFO) are either weight relieving or non-weight relieving calipers (Figs 3.28 to 3.31) It consists of the following parts:

- An upper end which may be made up of ring
- Cuff or bucket top
- It has two side bars or upright
- The knee joint
- The ankle joint
- A shoe
- Thigh
- Knee
- Calf bands

39b. What are the types of calipers?

Ans. Hip-Knee-Ankle-Foot Orthoses and Lumbosacral Hip-Knee-Ankle-Foot Orthoses.

A pelvic band may be attached to the KAFO with or without a hip joint to convert to a hip-knee-ankle-foot orthoses (HKAFO). And if this is extended upwards, a lumbosacral support is obtained converting it to a lumbosacral hip-knee-ankle- foot orthoses (LHKAFO).

The purpose of the pelvic band at the hip joint is to:

- Prevent development of a flexion deformity in polio, cerebral palsy.
- To increase the stability of spine.

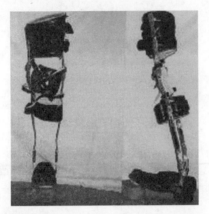

Fig. 3.28: KAFO (Double metal uprights)

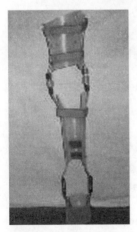 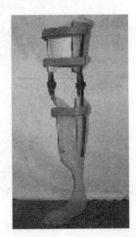

Fig. 3.29: KAFO (drop ring lock)   Fig. 3.30: KAFO (Plastic shell with metal uprights and drop lock joints

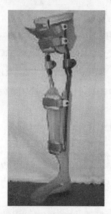

Fig. 3.31: KAFO (with offset knee joints)

ANKLE-FOOT ORTHOSES

Ankle-foot orthosis is a below knee orthosis in which the ankle joint can be controlled either by mechanical ankle joints or by heel straps (Figs 3.32 to 3.37).

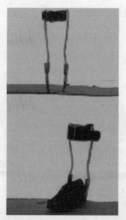

Fig. 3.32: AFO (Double metal upright)

39c. What are the uses of a caliper?
Ans. All the above lower limb orthoses so far mentioned are useful either to prevent or to correct deformities due to

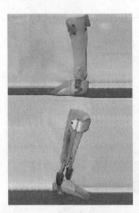

Fig. 3.33: Ankle-foot orthosis (Modular type)

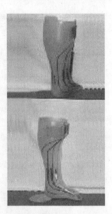

Fig. 3.34: AFO (Thermoplastic moulded)

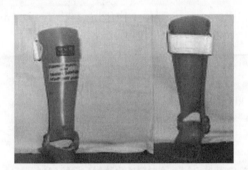

Fig. 3.35: AFO (Flesh colored plasticgelett joint with dorsiflexion assist

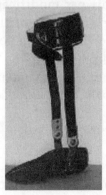

Fig. 3.36: AFO (Carbon plastic with foot plate)

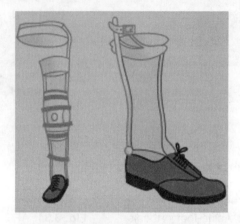

Fig. 3.37: AFO

polio, cerebral palsy, spina bifida, etc. They can be used either temporarily or permanently.

Rapid Recall Lower Limb Orthoses
- AFO—ankle foot orthoses.
- KAFO—knee-ankle-foot orthoses.
- HKAFO—hip knee-ankle-foot orthoses.
- THKAFO—trunk-hip-knee-ankle-foot orthoses.

FOOTWEAR AND ITS MODIFICATIONS

40. What are the footwear modifications?
Ans. The following are some of the modifications of footwear useful in the clinical situations mentioned below.
- *Rocker bar*: For hallux rigidus.
- *Outside heel float*: For lateral ligament injuries of the ankle.
- *Heel pad*: For heel pain.
- *Medial longitudinal arch support* (Fig. 3.39) To relieve pain, the following supports are used.
  - Valgus insole.
  - Thomas' heel (extension of medial aspect of the heel).
  - Filling of the medial half of the shank of the shoes (medial shank filler).

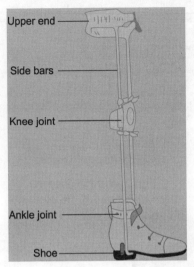

Fig. 3.38: KAFO

- *Metatarsal arch*: It is supported by the dome-shaped metatarsal bars.

- *More roomy footwear*: To accommodate deformed toes.

41. Name the different types of surgical footwears.

Ans. The different types of surgical footwears are mentioned in Table 3.4:

Table 3.4: Surgical footwears (Figs 3.39 to 3.49)

Footwear	Indications
Thomas' heel	Flat foot
Arch support	Flat foot
CTEV shoes	For CTEV
Heel pad	Calcaneal spur and plantar fasciitis
Metatarsal pad	For corns
Metatarsal bar	Metatarsalgia
Medial raise	Genu valgum
Lateral raise	Genu varum
Universal	For short leg
Upper limb orthosis	

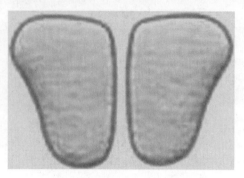

Fig. 3.39: Arch support

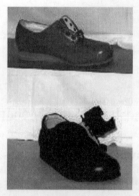

Fig. 3.40a: Blucher type Orthopedic shoe (top), Diabetes shoe (bottom)

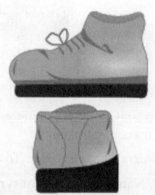

Fig. 3.40b: CTEV shoes

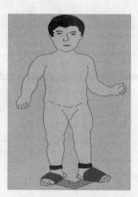

Fig. 3.41: Denis Browne splint

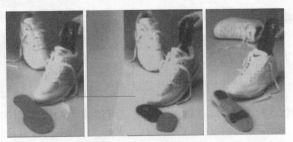

Fig. 3.42: Foot inserts

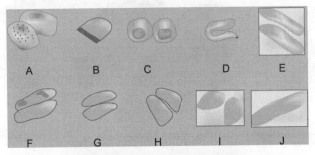

Figs 3.43A to J: Foot supports

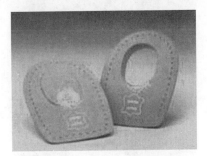

Fig. 3.44: Leather heel supports

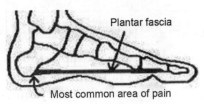

Fig. 3.45: Plantar fascia

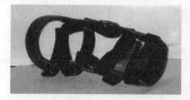

Fig. 3.46: Plaster shoes

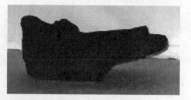

Fig. 3.47: Rocker shoe

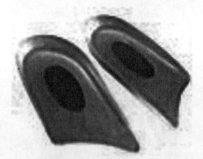

Fig. 3.48: Silicon heel

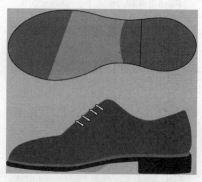

Fig. 3.49: UCBL heel insert and metatarsal bars

UPPER LIMB ORTHOSIS

42. Mention the role of upper limb orthosis.

Ans. Upper limb orthosis ranges from a simple splint to the very complex varieties which are manufactured to the following basic requirements:

- Limitation of movements could be either total or partial.
- Exercise of muscles and joints range against energy storing devices such as springs or elastics.
- Replacement of paralysed muscles using similar devices.
- Preventive deformity control.

43. Name the common braces used in orthopedic practice.
Ans. In the following are the commonly used orthopedic braces (Figs 3.50 to 3.55):

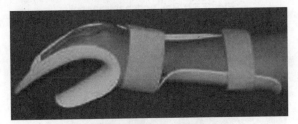

Fig. 3.50: Resting hand splint

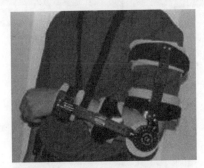

Fig. 3.51: Bledsoe arm brace

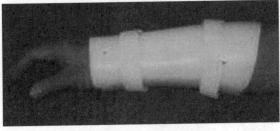

Fig. 3.52: Ulnar gutter splint

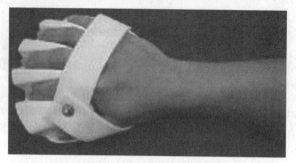

Fig. 3.53: Ball antispasticity splint

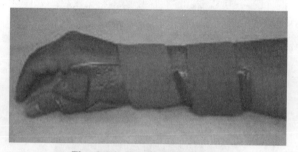

Fig. 3.54: Thumb spical splint

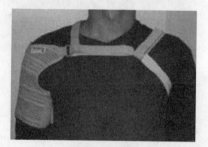

Fig. 3.55: Hemiplegic brace

Braces

- A—Knee support cap
- B—Ankle supports
- C—Elbow support
- D—Cervical collar
- E—Sacrolumbar support

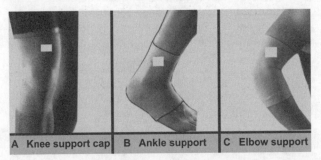

A Knee support cap | B Ankle support | C Elbow support

Fig. 3.56: Joint elastic supports

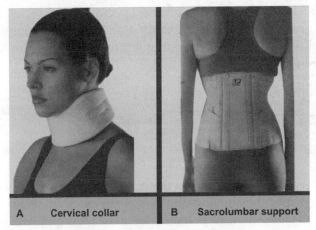

A Cervical collar | B Sacrolumbar support

Fig. 3.57

44. What are the uses of the above braces?

Ans. The braces have the following functions:

- Provides support
- Provides pair relief
- Allows protected function of the affected parts
- Provides psychological boost to the patients.

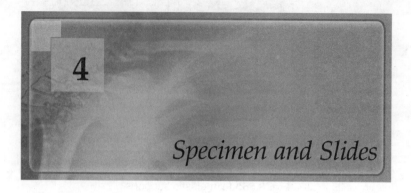

4

Specimen and Slides

This chapter deals with typical specimen and slides which are given in the practical examinations for the students. This book is useful for exam going students and also for young orthopedic surgeons.

Tumor Disorders	
• Osteogenic sarcoma	• Ewing's sarcoma
• Chondrosarcoma	• Benign bone tumors
• GCT	• Infective disorders
	• Metabolic and inflammatory disorders

Here you need to identify the bony specimen and you need to identify their histopathological slides.

TUMOR DISORDERS

OSTEOGENIC SARCOMA

Osteogenic sarcoma is a highly malignant primary bone tumor. Here tumor cells invariably form a neoplastic osteoid, bone, or both. It arises from a common multifactorial mesenchymal tissue and hence the tumor could be either *fibroblastic, osteoblastic* or *chondroblastic*. This is the most frequent primary bone tumor next only to multiple myeloma. It is common in the second decade, rare below 10 years of age, 75 percent of the cases are seen below the age of 25. Male preponderance, when found in females it starts at an early age. *Incidence* is 1/75,000 population.

Site ninety percent of the tumor occurs in the metaphysial region of the ends of long bones. It has a predilection around the knee and upper humerus. It may affect the jaws in the aged.

Pathology

The tumor could be either osteoblastic, chondroblastic or fibroblastic. Consequently the tumor may be osteosclerotic or osteolytic. Most common tumor is both a combination of osteosclerotic and osteolytic variety.

Gross the tumor is more commonly situated in metaphysis of a large long bone. It is a large tumor with areas of destruction gives an appearance of *leg of mutton.* The consistency ranges from stony hard to soft. The color of the tumor could be w*hite* if the tumor is *fibroblastic,* y*ellowish white* if os*teoblastic, bluish white* if the tumor is c*artilaginous.* At the areas of rapid growth, there are necrotic foci, cavitations and hemorrhage. *Sunray* appearance is seen in the subperiosteal space due to bone deposition along the vessels. *Codman's triangle* is a reactive bone formation parallel to the bone and is triangular in shape.

Histology: Small spindle cells with hyper chromatic nuclei are seen. The shape may be round, cuboidal or columnar. Cells are pleomorphic in nature. Large spindle-shaped cells are rare. Giant cells are often present. Matrix may be myxomatous, cartilaginous or osseous. Areas of hemorrhage may be present. Normally when the bone forms an osteoid tissue, it is preceded by the stage of chondrification. *Neoplastic or tumor osteoid formed from the primitive malignant cells skip the stage of chondrification and form the ossified tissue directly without any intervening stage of chondrification.*

Classification: Primary and Secondary

Clinical features the patient usually presents with pain. Patient complains of tired feeling and limp. General condition is good till the late stages. Pyrexia is seen with increased WBCs. Patient is usually anemic than cachectic. Swelling develops later and the skin over the tumor is stretched, shiny and mobile. Local temperature is increased, consistency of the tumor is variable, dilated veins are present (and is evident at an early stage). Pathological fracture is not typical of osteogenic sarcoma since the swelling and pain keeps the patient off his or her feet. The nearest joint may show pain and effusion. Joint movements may be unimpaired but there could be a mechanical block caused by the tumor bulk. Neurovascular structures could be compressed.

Treatment: General Principles

1. Early radical amputation is done to remove the primary tumor.
2. An attempt is made to prevent metastasis or control it if it has already formed by preoperative irradiation, chemotherapy or both.
3. Resection of large pulmonary metastasis is carried out.

Surgery: Early *and radical ablation* is the surgical procedure of choice. Having first established the diagnosis by biopsy, the level of amputation is determined after carrying out the various investigations mentioned above. Surgery is done at the *earliest* possible time.

Remember

Characteristic facts of osteogenic sarcoma
- Highly malignant bone tumor.
- Arises from multipotent cells.
- Most frequent primary bone tumor next only to multiple myeloma.
- Seventy-five percent are below 25 years of age.
- Ninety percent occur in the metaphysis.
- Neoplastic osteoid is always present.
- Both osteosclerotic and osteolytic variety is the most common.
- Leg of mutton appearance.
- Spindle cells.
- No giant cells.
- Pain is the first symptom.
- Skin is stretched shiny, dilated veins are present.
- Pathological fractures are not common.
- Eighty percent has blood spread.

- Sunray appearance and Codman's triangle are special X-ray features.
- Multipronged approach gives better survival rate.

Highlights

- Metaphyseal tumor
- Hemorrhagic areas
- Cortex broken
- Epiphyseal plate croded

Histology

- Proliferating spindle cells (that directly produce osteoid or immature bone).
- High-grade anaplasia (Marked pleomorphosis, chromatin abnormalities, prominent nucleoli, atypical mitotis).

Treatment

- Highly sensitive to chemotherapy for 8–12 weeks.
- Followed by conservative surgery or amputation.
- Again a session of postoperative chemotherapy.

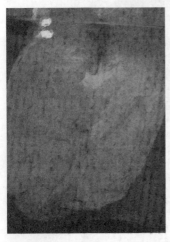 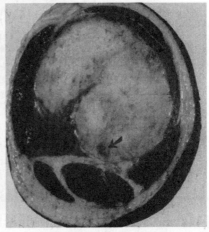

Fig. 4.1: Osteogenic sarcoma (Mounted specimen)

Fig. 4.2: Osteosarcoma

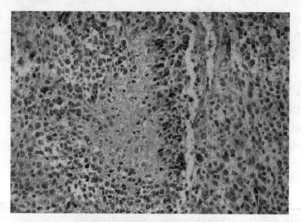

Fig. 4.3: Osteosarcoma slide

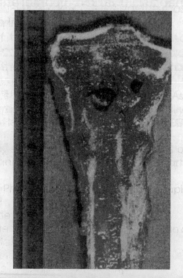

Fig. 4.4: Osteosarcoma surgical specimen

CHONDROSARCOMA

This is *second* in frequency to osteosarcoma. It arises from the cartilage cells. It is a malignant but *slow* growing tumor. It has a long history and a better prognosis. Unlike osteogenic sarcoma, there is *no neoplastic osteoid formation and alkaline phosphatase is usually not raised.* It ranges from being locally aggressive to high-grade malignancy. Primary/secondary Secondary tumors develop when benign cartilaginous tumors are irradiated. It is common at the sites of proximal femur, humerus, ribs, and scapula, in nominate bones, rare in hands and feet except in calcaneus, and occur in pelvis or upper femora. Males are more commonly affected than females. Twenty to sixty years, rare below 20 years, peak in the sixth decade.

Symptoms: The duration of symptoms are usually less than 2 years in 75 percent of the cases and less than 5 years in the remaining 25 percent. Pain is usually not a prominent feature unlike osteogenic sarcoma. The central tumor remains entirely asymptomatic until it has eroded and penetrated the cortex or caused a pathological fracture. A palpable firm mass attached to the bone is the common physical sign. The tumor may assume large proportion.

Low and medium grade lesions require wide excision, e.g. forequarter amputation (Thikor-Linberg) for the shoulder girdle; hindquarter amputation for the pelvic girdle.

High-grade lesions require radical marginal excision role of systemic chemotherapy in chondrosarcoma is controversial.

Palliative radiotherapy is indicated when the tumor cannot be resected because of its enormous size or if the tumor is present in inaccessible region.

Quick facts in Chondrosarcoma

- Second in frequency to osteosarcoma.
- No neoplastic osteoid.
- Long history.
- Pain is not a prominent feature.
- X-ray—*popcorn* appearance.
- Wide excision is the treatment of choice.
- Better survival rate.

Highlights

- Central type (located within the medullary cavity of the lower end of femur).
- Peripheral type (located in the upper end of femur).
- Slow growing
- Assumes large proportions.

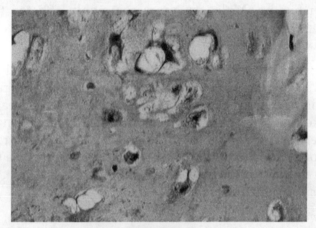

Fig. 4.5: Chondrosarcoma slide

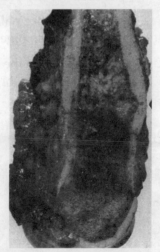

Fig. 4.6: Chondrosarcoma specimen

Histological Highlights
- Low cellularity
- Low cytonuclear atypia
- Less multinucleated cells
- Chrondroid matrix
- Mitoses absent

Features are suggestive of grade I chondrosarcoma. As the grade increases the cellularity increases with nuclear polymorphism and muco-myxoid degeneration of the matrix.

Treatment
- Highly resistant to chemotherapy and radiotherapy.
- Surgery is the treatment of choice.

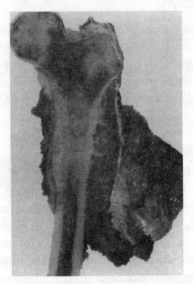

Fig. 4.7: Chondrosarcoma specimen of femur

GIANT CELL TUMOR (GCT)

Benign giant cell tumor is an osteolytic tumor arising from the *epiphysis* and is common in young adults. Though it is benign, it is *locally* malignant. The presence of *tumor giant cells* is the hallmark of this tumor. The male: female ratio is 1.5:1. It is common between 15 and 35 years 80% occur in more than 20 years of age and the average age group is 35. Areas affected are asymmetric portions of the epiphysis of long bones. About 75 percent of GCT occurs in lower end of femur, upper end of tibia, fibula and the distal end of radius.

Pathology

Gross: The tumor consists of ragged, friable, bleeding tissue filled with old or fresh blood clots with various sized cysts and cavities. Color varies from red to brown. Epiphyseal end of the bone is distorted. Tumor extension into the joint cavity is usually not seen and there is no evidence of periosteal reaction.

Microscopy: The tumor is encompassed by a fibrous capsule at the periphery. Presence of abundant tumor giant cells is quite characteristic. These cells are characterized by their larger size, multiple nuclei more than 150 in number, which are distributed through out the cell. Appearance of spindle cells indicates *malignant* potential.

Clinical Features

The course of the tumor is chronic. Unlike osteogenic sarcoma, pain is not the presenting feature but trauma is, the patient complains of swelling which is situated on one side of the bone. Skin over the tumor is stretched but there are no dilated veins. Tenderness is moderate or absent, *egg shell crackling* sensation may be present or absent. Limitation of joint movements is not seen till the late stages. There is no increase in joint fluid and the joint is rarely invaded. Pathological fracture is a late feature.

MALIGNANT GCT

Primary this develops as a frank sarcomatous lesion.

Secondary this develops at the site of previously treated GCT.

Treatment of GCT: Principles of tumor treatment

- The tumor is invasive and aggressive.
- It commonly recurs, may become malignant after unsuccessful removal.
- Recurrence is treated with *en bloc* excision.
- *En block* excision is also indicated if the tumor has eroded the cortex and extended into the soft tissues.

Irradiation therapy induces malignant change if it is given to the benign lesion. Megavoltage therapy is permissible only for inaccessible lesions located in the spine, sacrum, pelvis, etc. The recommended dosage is 1500 to 5000 rads for 5 to 6 weeks.

Quick facts of GCT

- Locally malignant.
- Affects young adults.
- Arises from the epiphysis.
- Giant cells are characteristic.
- Egg shell crackling may be present.
- Soap-bubble appearance is characteristic.
- *En bloc* excision and reconstruction is the surgical method of choice.
- One-third is benign, one-third is locally malignant and one-third is malignant.

Highlights

- A well-defined eccenteric lesion involving epiphysis and metaphysis.
- Bubbly appearance.

Histological Highlights

- Tumoral spindle cells (neoplastic).
- Rounded mononuclear cells.
- Osteoclastic type of giant cells.
- Small blood vessels.

Treatment

Surgery is the treatment of choice. The procedure of choice is 'Excision'.

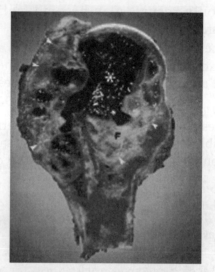

Fig. 4.8: GCT proximal humerus (Surgical specimen)

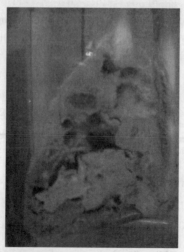

Fig. 4.9: Giant cell tumor lower end of radius (Mounted specimen)

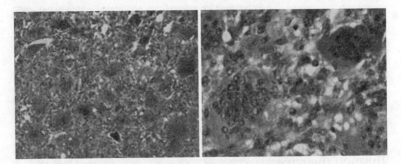

Fig. 4.10: Giant cell tumor slide

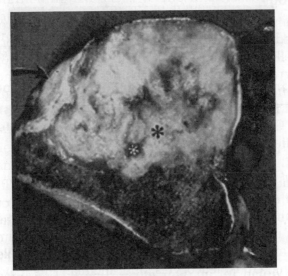

Fig. 4.11: Malignant GCT

EWING'S SARCOMA

Ewing's sarcoma was first described by Ewing in the year 1928. This is a rare primary malignant bone tumor (10–14% of all malignant bone tumors) affecting children. It is a lethal tumor with a poor 5-year survival rate. *Age* persons commonly affected are four to twenty-five years of age group (about 80%). *Sex* more common in males. *Site* long bones affected are femur, tibia, fibula and humerus in that order. About 20 percent of tumors are seen in flat bones. *Location* diaphysis of the long bones is commonly affected.

Pathology

Gross: It is a grayish white tumor encapsulated by fibrous tissue. It may contain hemorrhagic foci and areas of cystic formation. From the medulla, it reaches to the surface through the haversian canals.

Histology

The tumor is very *cellular.* The cells may be small, round or polyhedral in shape and may be arranged as cords or sheets. Intercellular substance is minimal. Necrosis is common. Cells are arranged round the vessels justifying the term *perithelioma.* Many tumors show *Rosette* formation with central fibril. *Pseudo rosettes* are more common (no central fibril). Giant cells are not found and there is no new bone formation.

Clinical Features

Patient presents with pain, which is intermittent in nature. The pain is worse at night. The tumor is fixed to the bone, skin is red, dilated veins may be present. Some times the tumor may present with constitutional symptoms like fever, sweating, chills, leucocytes, and anemia. This may create confusion as it mimics acute osteomyelitis.

Biopsy is necessary for diagnosis

Recommended treatment: This tumor is highly radiosensitive, disappears with radiation only to recur (melts like snow). Hence a combination of local radiotherapy with systemic chemotherapy brings down the recurrence rate dramatically. However, even this treatment has a recurrence rate of 20 to 30 percent and because of the possibility of radiation-induced sarcomas; surgical resection for the control of the primary lesion is being used. The surgery planned is conservative in nature and aims at limb preservation.

Effective chemotherapy is given using newer chemotherapeutic drugs like ifosfamide, cisplatinum, epipodophyllin toxin for a short period of time.

Radiation is the mainstay of local treatment especially in axial skeleton. Dose required is high 4000 rads for the entire limb and 1000 rads as boost to the tumor.

Surgery conservative surgery like debulking of the tumors or limb preservation surgery has a role.

Quick facts of Ewing's sarcoma
- Rare primary malignant tumor.
- Common between 5 and 15 years.
- Tumor of the diaphysis.
- Clinically may mimic acute osteomyelitis.
- X-ray shows moth-eaten appearance and onion peel appearance.
- Tumor is highly cellular.
- Highly radiosensitive (melts like snow).
- High rate of recurrence.
- Combination of radiotherapy, chemotherapy and surgery has improved two-year survival rate.

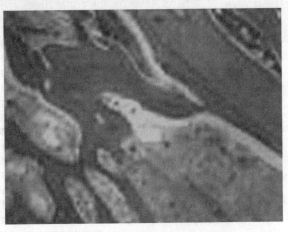

Fig. 4.12: Ewing's sarcoma slide

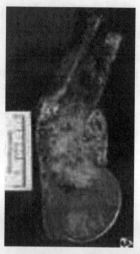

Fig. 4.13: Ewing specimen

BENIGN BONE TUMORS

CHONDROBLASTOMA

This is a highly cellular, vascular, and cartilaginous benign bone tumor of the cancellous bone. Here the cancellous bone is destroyed and multiple calcium deposits are usually found within the tumor. *Age* 10 to 20 years. *sex* male preponderance. *sites* epiphyseal ends of long bones are commonly affected. *Symptoms* the patient may present with pain, swelling, joint effusion, etc.

Radiology

Radiographic features of the tumor are areas of rarefaction at epiphysis, eccentric position of the tumor, thin cortex and mottled areas of calcification.

Treatment

This consists of curettage and bone grafting if the lesion is small, excision in bigger tumors. If it is accidentally irradiated it may turn malignant. Recurrence rate after excision is 25%.

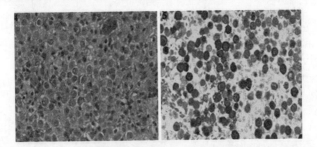

Fig. 4.14: Chondroblastoma

CHONDROMA (Enchondroma, Chondromyxoma)

This is a benign cartilaginous tumor centrally located when it occurs in phalanges and humerus. It causes destruction of the cancellous bone and has a potential for undergoing malignant change, especially when it is situated in the long bones.

- Age—10 to 50 years.
- Site—metaphysis is usually involved. It is common in the phalanges of hand (little finger common) and feet. Innominate and long bones may also be involved.
- Symptoms are practically none. There may be slight pain and the phalanx may be enlarged.
- The course of the tumor is very slow.

Treatment

Curettage is done and the wall is cauterized if the tumor is small. The surgery done in cases of large tumors is excision and removal of the capsule to prevent recurrence. Radical resection is done for tumors of long bones and pelvis. *Recurrence is common with chondromas of the long bones.*

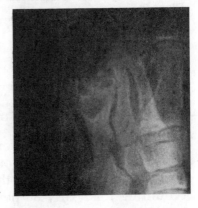

Fig. 4.15: Chondromyxoid fibroma

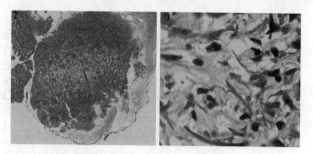

Fig. 4.16: Chondromyxoid fibroma slide

INFECTIVE DISORDERS

CHRONIC OSTEOMYELITIS

Osteomyelitis is defined as a suppurative process of the bone caused by pyogenic organisms or simply a pyogenic infection of the cancellous portion of the bone. Two types are described based on duration of symptoms as acute or chronic. Any osteomyelitis lasting for more than three weeks is termed as chronic. *Sequestra is a dead bone within a living bone and is defined as an infected granulation tissue. The inflammatory foci are surrounded by sclerotic bone supplied with blood and covered by periosteum, scarred muscle and subcutaneous tissues.*

Disease		Type of sequestra
TB osteomyelitis	→	Sandy/feathery
Actinomycosis	→	Black
Pin tract infection	→	Ring
Chronic osteomyelitis in children	→	Diaphyseal

TUBERCULOSIS SPINE (Known after Sir Percivall Pott)

This is the most common form of skeletal tuberculosis constituting about 50 percent of all cases. Spinal tuberculosis commonly affects the lower thoracic and lumbar vertebra accounting for nearly 80 percent of the cases. Sites of involvement within the vertebra. It is observed that spinal tuberculosis could start in any of the part of the vertebra (95% anterior; 5% posterior elements).

Sequences of Pathological Events

As mentioned earlier due to primary foci in the lungs, lymph nodes or abdomen, bacillemia develops and the organisms reach the spine through the Batson plexus. Tuberculous endarteritis which develops following the infection results in marrow devitalization. Later on the tubercular follicle develops. Lamellae are destroyed due to hyperemia causing osteoporosis. As a result of this the vertebral body gets easily compressed. In the thoracic vertebrae because of the normal kyphotic curve, anterior wedge compression is more common. In the lordotic cervical and lumbar vertebra, wedging is minimal.

This non-pyogenic infection results in formation of cold abscess which penetrates the epiphyseal cortex and involves the adjacent disk and the vertebra. It may also spread beneath the anterior longitudinal ligament and reach the neighboring

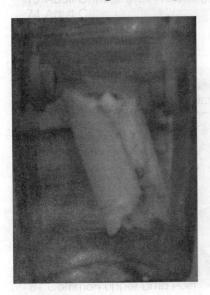 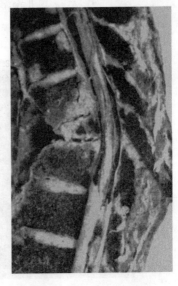

Fig. 4.17 Sequestrum   **Fig. 4.18** TB spine specimen

vertebra. When it spreads posteriorly it may cause pressure on the spinal cord which is more common in the thoracic area as the spinal canal is small here. The posterior longitudinal ligament limits the spread of sequestra and bone fragments into the joints. Sometimes the cold abscess may penetrate the anterior longitudinal ligament and migrate along the *lines of least resistance* (i.e. along the fascial planes, blood vessels, nerves) and may get manifested elsewhere far away from the original lesion. Healing in the spine is by bony fusion.

METABOLIC AND INFLAMMATORY DISORDERS

MONOSODIUM URATE ARTHROPATHY (GOUT)

This is known as *gout* and may manifest itself as *acute* or *chronic*. It is usually monoarticular and the first metatarsophalangeal joint is the most common site of involvement. Ankle, knee, wrist, fingers and elbow are other joints affected. *Distal and lower extremity joints are involved more often.* Gout is usually associated with hyperuricemia and may be associated with hypertension, obesity and atherosclerosis. Synovial fluid study is done under polarised

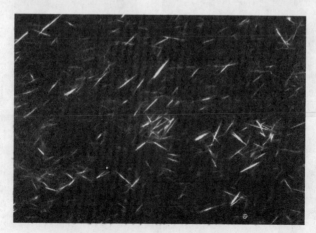

Fig. 4.19: Crystalline arthropathy (gout)

microscopy for the presence of monosodium urate crystals. This is the most important diagnostic method.

RHEUMATOID ARTHRITIS

Rheumatoid arthritis is the *most common* inflammatory disease of the joints. It is a systemic disease of young and middle-aged adults characterized by proliferative and destructive changes in synovial membrane, periarticular structures, skeletal muscles and perineural sheaths. Eventually joints are destroyed, fibrosed or ankylosed. *It is a widespread vasculitis of the small arterioles.*

Pathology

Due to the synthesis of autoantibodies, against unknown antigenic agents in the synovium, primary synovitis sets in. This primary synovitis gives rise to pannus, which in turn forms the villus. This villus migrates towards the joint causing its destruction and ankylosis, fibrous in the early stages followed by bony ankylosis in the late stages.

Microscopy

It reveals rheumatoid units, which are an area of fibrinoid necrosis surrounded by fibroblasts, arranged radially and it

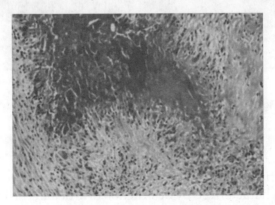

Fig. 4.20: Rheumatoid nodule

is surrounded by a fibrous capsule. This rheumatoid unit is found in the muscle, vessels, nerves, synovium, etc.

OSTEOPOROSIS

It is a generic term referring to a state of decreased mass per unit volume of a normally mineralized bone due to loss of bone proteins. It is the most common skeletal disorder in the world, next only to arthritis. In osteoporosis, there is a long latent period before clinical symptoms develop. Most prevalent complications are fractures of vertebral bodies, ribs, proximal femur, humerus, distal radius with minimal trauma. Most common cause is involutional bone loss in perimenopausal age group. In osteoporosis decreased density is due to deficiency of protein matrix in which calcium is laid down, here rate of bone resorption is greater than bone formation, most commonly it is due to aging process but the most common cause is involutional bone loss in perimenopausal women.

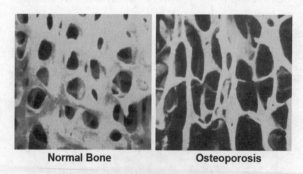

Normal Bone   **Osteoporosis**

Fig. 4.21: Normal bone (left), osteoporotic bone (right)

OSTEOARTHRITIS

It is defined as a degenerative, non-inflammatory joint disease characterized by destruction of articular cartilage and formation of new bone at the joint surfaces and margins.

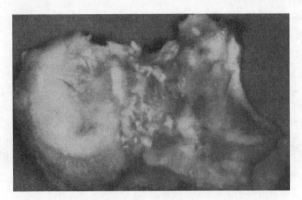

Fig. 4.22: Osteoarthritic cartilage specimen

There are two varieties, primary and secondary. The former is more common. Knee joint is affected more often than any other joint.

Sequence of Pathological Events in Osteoarthritis

Fibrillation due to loss of water of the weight-bearing articular cartilage is seen in early stages of the disease followed by complete loss of articular cartilage. This puts enormous pressure on the underlying bone which causes sclerosis and later eburnation. Cysts may develop in the subchondral area due to micro fractures that degenerate. New bone formation takes place and results in osteophyte formation. Synovial inflammation and capsular thickening causes effusion and joint stiffness.

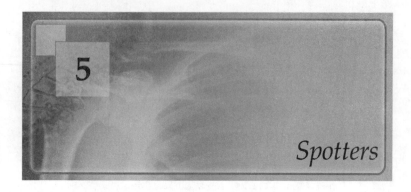

5

Spotters

This is again not a feature in most of the university exams but may figure in National board exams. Here you are required to make a spot diagnosis without taking the history, examination of the patient or looking into the X-rays. Here you are only getting to see but not talk or touch the patient. Hence it is a test of your **visual diagnostic** skills. Classical cases will be kept and more often than not you will find no difficulty in spotting the diagnosis. However there could be some overlap sometimes between the spotters and short cases. For example, a wrist drop case could be either kept as a spotter or given as a short case.

It is an interesting part of the examination whenever given and like an MCQ question you may score a quick and full mark on spotting a case correctly. If given a chance go for it with full gutso and score as much as possible.

LIKELY QUESTIONS

- What is your diagnosis?
- Why do you say so?
- What are the clinical features?
- What are the relevant investigations?
- What is the differential diagnosis?
- Name the treatment options.
- What are the likely complications?

This and many more could be the likely questions after you spot the case correctly.

CONGENITAL ANOMALIES

CONGENITAL HAND DEFORMITIES

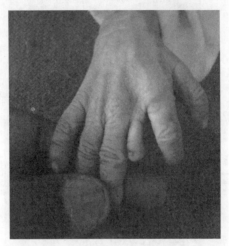

Fig. 5.1: Accessory fingers

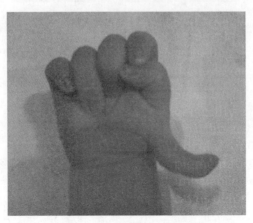

Fig. 5.2: Accessory thumb

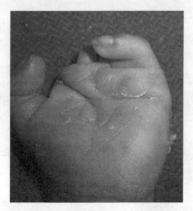

Fig. 5.3: Hypoplasia phalanges

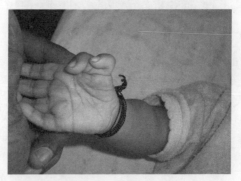

Fig. 5.4: Polydactyly

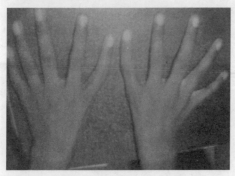

Fig. 5.5: Triphalangeal thumb

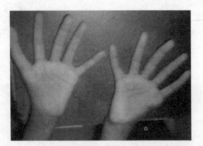

Fig. 5.6: Triphalangeal thumb

CONGENITAL FOOT AND LOWER LIMB DEFORMITIES

CONGENITAL VERTICAL TALUS
(Popularly known as Rocker Bottom Foot)

Normally talus is placed horizontally in the hindfoot. Sometimes due to a congenital abnormality, it may remain vertical. A vertical talus reverses the normal concave arch with the abnormal convex arch (likened to the *Rocker Bottom* of an easy chair). Additionally the foot may be in severe valgus. X-ray of the foot clinches the diagnosis. The navicle instead of being in front of the talus sits on top of it.

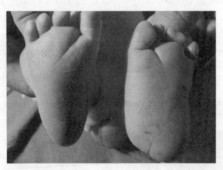

Fig. 5.7: Rocker bottom foot (Congenital vertical talus)

Pes Planus

This refers to loss of medial-longitudinal arch of the foot. Medial arch is obliterated, navicular bone is prominent, and fingers cannot be inserted under the arch, sole of the foot. Area of weight bearing increases and may show increased callosity.

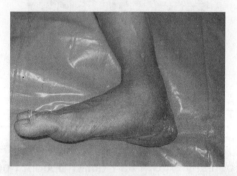

Fig. 5.8: Flat foot

Pes Cavus

Pes cavus is a deformity characterized by an excessively high longitudinal arch that results from an equinus position of the forefoot in relation to the hind foot. *In this condition finger can be slipped under the navicular bone and it penetrates a distance of greater than 2 cm from the vertical edge of the foot.* Clinical features consist of high medial longitudinal arch, first metatarsal drop and pronation, tight plantar fascia, cock-up deformities of all the toes at the MTP joints, varus heel, and clawing of the toes (late feature).

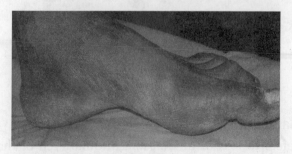

Fig. 5.9: Pes cavus

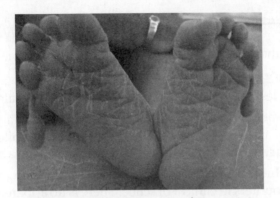

Fig. 5.10: Polydactyly v

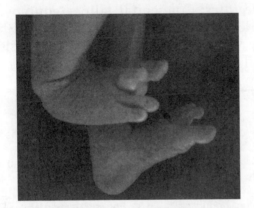

Fig. 5.11: Syndactyly

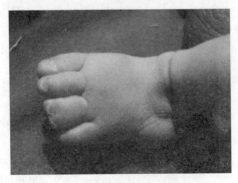

Fig. 5.12: Syndactyly

CONGENITAL TALIPES EQUINOVARUS (CTEV) FOOT

This is the most common congenital foot disorder.

Incidence is 1.2/1000 live births.

Sex: Males are more commonly affected than females.

Etiology of CTEV: This could be primary or secondary in the primary variety exact cause is the unknown, while in the secondary variety the causes could be polio, spine bifida.

Idiopathic CTEV: This is the most common type of CTEV one encounters in clinical practice. There is no apparent cause and hence, various theories are proposed.

Clinical features: Congenital talipes equinovarus is a grotesque looking deformity of the foot. In idiopathic variety deformity is the only complaint. The diagnosis is fairly simple and straightforward. *Five classical primary deformities*

Clubfoot Complex	
Primary deformities ↓	**Secondary deformities** ↓
1. Equinus	1. Foot size is decreased to 50%
2. Varus	2. Medial border is concave, lateral
3. Cavus	border is convex
4. Forefoot adduction	3. Forefoot is plantar flexed upon
5. Internal tibial torsion	hindfoot
	4. Skin is stretched over the dorsum
Late changes	of the foot
1. Degeneration of joints	5. Callosities are present over the
2. Fusion of joints	dorsum of the foot
	6. Stumbling gait
	7. Hypotrophic anterior tibial artery
	8. Atrophy of muscles in anterior or
	posterior compartments of the leg
	9. Tight plantar fascia and tendo-Achilles on attempting correction.
	10. Transverse skin crease.
	11. Heel is small and is impalpable.

are seen and in response to this, secondary deformities develop. These primary and secondary deformities together form the clubfoot complex. A detailed examination of the foot is necessary to detect the full spectrum of deformities in CTEV.

With advancing age, the cosmetically unsightly clubfoot starts posing functional problems like altered gait (stumbling gait) callosities, degeneration and arthritic changes in the ankle and foot joints. Correction is a must to restore normalcy.

In other varieties of CTEV, clinical features peculiar to the etiological factors can be elicited.

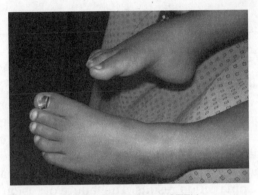

Fig. 5.13: Unilateral CTEV

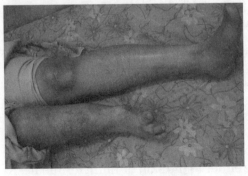

Fig. 5.14: Gross shortening

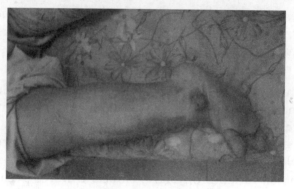

Fig. 5.15: Deformity closer view

CONGENITAL SPINE DEFORMITIES

SPINA BIFIDA

Embryo logically the mesoderm around the notochord develops into vertebral body. The vertebral arch is formed by two projections from the vertebral body which grow backward enclosing in between them the neural canal and fuse in the center. The fusion starts at the thoracic region and extends up and down. When these vertebral arches err in fusion, spina bifida results. The failure of fusion could be limited, only to the spinous process resulting in spina bifida occulta, the most common variety or the entire vertebral arch including the neural elements may fail to fuse giving rise to the rare variety of spina bifida aperta.

Spina bifida occulta: This is the most common variety and is generally mild. Lumbosacral spine and the first sacral vertebra are commonly affected. The overlying skin may be normal or there may be presence of a tuft of hair, pigmentation, lipoma, dimple, etc. There may be muscle imbalance in the lower limbs resulting in equinovarus or cavus deformity of the foot due to tethering of the cord by a membrane either to the skin or filum terminale. Rarely there could be a bifid cord.

Spina bifida aperta here the defect involves the vertebral arches, skin, meninges and cord. The following varieties are described:

a. *Meningocele* in which there is protrusion of the meninges.
b. *Myelomeningocele* in which there is protrusion of meninges and cord.
c. *Syringomyelocele* in which central canal of the cord is dilated and the cord is protruded.
d. *Myelocele* in which the central cord remains unfused and exposed.

Next to spina bifida occulta, myelocele is the next common variety. Most of the cases of spina bifida aperta are either stillborn or die within few days of birth. The surviving children may suffer from severe orthopedic deformities, bladder and bowel incontinence and foot deformities.

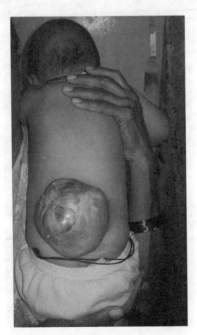

Fig. 5.16: Myelomeningocele

SCOLIOSIS

By definition, Scoliosis is a lateral curvature of the spine in the upright position. The lateral curvature is usually accompanied by some rotational deformity. Though idiopathic scoliosis can occur at any age, it usually appears clinically between 10 and 13 years. It is more common in

Quick facts
- Scoliosis is lateral curvature of the spine.
- Idiopathic variety accounts for 90% of cases.
- Female preponderance.
- X-ray is the only definite documentation of curve size and progression.
- The most important aspect of treatment is early detection.
- Curves < 20° need observation.
- Curves > 20° require treatment.
- Curves between 20 and 40° can be treated by Milwaukee brace, which has to be worn 23 hrs per day for a period of at least two years.
- Curves > 40° need surgical correction and fusion.

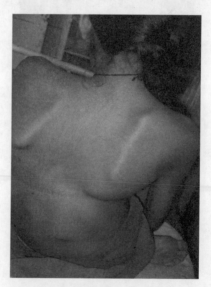

Fig. 5.17: Kyphoscoliosis

females. The disease is usually asymptomatic and is usually accidentally discovered. The diagnosis is usually made on routine physical examination especially during medical examination at schools. Look for different varieties of curves. In long-standing cases, patients may complain of pain, there could be impaired lung function and rarely neurological deficits.

OTHER ANOMALIES

MUCOPOLYSACCHARIDOSIS

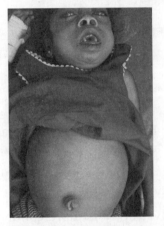

Fig. 5.18: MPS type I

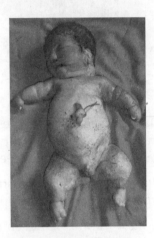

Fig. 5.19: Phocomelia

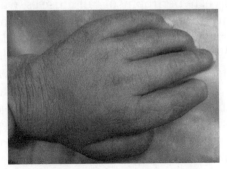

Fig. 5.20: MPS type I

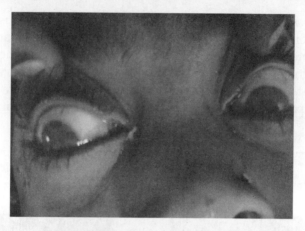

Fig. 5.21: MPS type I

DEVELOPMENTAL ANOMALIES

Muscular dystrophies: These are difficult problems to treat and the cause is usually not known. A few important muscular dystrophies in each variety is described below.

Duchenne's muscular dystrophy: This is the most common type of muscular dystrophy encountered.

Clinical features: Duchenne's dystrophy is more common in boys. This consists of delayed walking, abnormal gait and multiple falls (in less than 3 years child does). Gowers' sign is positive, hypertrophy of calf muscles, waddling gait, increased lumbar lordosis and weakness of shoulder muscles. Serrati, pectorals, deltoid, latissimus dorsi, biceps, triceps and brachialis muscles are weak. In lower limbs weakness of hip flexors, evertors of feet, tibialis anterior are seen, ocular, pharyngeal and masticatory muscles are never involved. Knee jerk is absent earlier than ankle jerk. Tendo-Achilles contractures appear first, later hamstrings, hip flexors and elbow follow. Intellectual impairment is present. Death below 16 years is due to respiratory infection or cardiac failure.

GOWERS' DISEASE

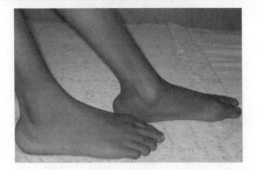

Fig. 5.22: Foot deformities

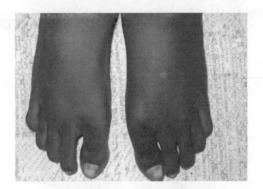

Fig. 5.23: Forefoot deformities

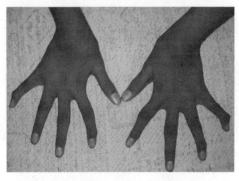

Fig. 5.24: Hand deformities

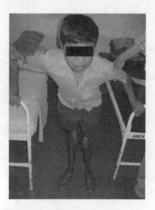

Fig. 5.25: Posture and gait

MORQUIO'S DISEASE

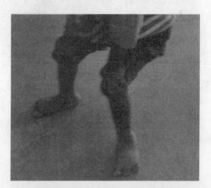

Fig. 5.26: Posture and gait

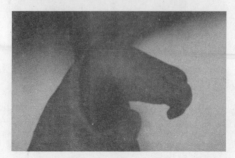

Fig. 5.27: Deformed hand

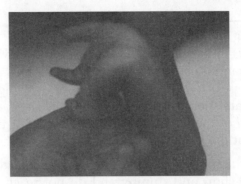

Fig. 5.28: Hypermobile joints

PAGET'S DISEASE

Paget's disease is seen after 40 years of age and is more common in males. There is impairment in the bone resorption and bone formation due to defective osteoclastic functions. As a result of this bone gets thickened and bent more so the tibia. Bone is soft in the initial stages and dense later. The affected bones are thickened and bent. Patient complains of dull pain and deformities.

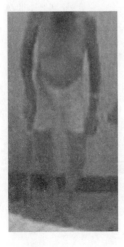

Fig. 5.29: Clinical picture

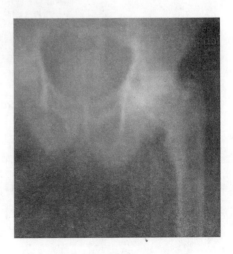

Fig. 5.30: X-ray of the hip

ACHONDROPLASIA

It is a defect in the enchondral ossification of the bone, with the membranous ossification being normal. This is the most common type of dwarfism one encounters in clinical practice The limbs are short and the head is big, because, along with the growth of the limbs, growth of the base of the skull is affected but the membranous bones of the vault escape.

Clinical features: The patient is a short-limbed dwarf. The fingers are short and stumpy and do not reach below the upper one-third of the thigh as he stands. Patient can kiss his toes with the knees straight. Head is large, nose is

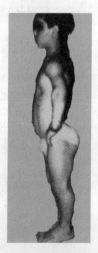

Fig. 5.31: Achondroplasia

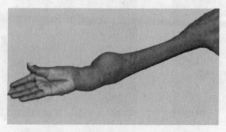

Fig. 5.32: Pseudarthrosis forearm

flattened but the length of the trunk may be normal and occasionally may show kyphoscoliosis or lordosis. Cervical lordosis and increased lumbar lordosis develop in the later stages of the disease. The intelligence and sexual developments are normal.

OSTEOGENESIS IMPERFECTA

It is a hereditary condition characterized by *fragility of bones, deafness, blue sclera, laxity of joints and a tendency to improve with age.* It is a disease of the mesodermal tissues with deposition of normal collagen in bone, skin, sclera and dentine.

Etiology the etiological factors could be heredity, Mendelian recessive—in prenatal cases, and Mendelian dominant—in postnatal cases.

Pathogenesis and pathology Primary defect is failure of osteoblast formation during enchondral ossification; osteoid formation does not take place.

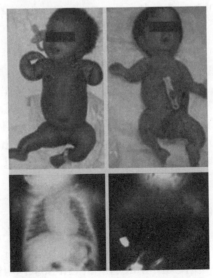

Fig. 5.33: Osteogenesis imperfecta

Clinical features patient presents with blue sclera, dentino-genesis imperfecta and generalized osteoporosis. Blue sclera is seen only in 92 percent of cases, while the other two features are seen in almost all cases. Osteoporosis gives rise to bowing and multiple fractures. Fractures are usually due to trivial trauma but surprisingly heal well. Other features include: deafness due to otosclerosis, laxity of joints, dwarfism, broad skull, poorly calcified decidual teeth but permanent teeth are normal and the blood chemistry is normal.

INFLAMMATORY DISORDERS

ANKYLOSING SPONDYLITIS
(Marie-Strümpell Diseases)

Definition

This is a chronic progressive inflammatory disease of the sacroiliac joints and the axial skeleton.

Causes

Causes are unknown. It is found to be strongly associated with HLA-B27 genetic marker is about 85 percent.

Age/sex: Common in young male adults (M: F = 10:1). In the 15–30 years age group.

Pathology

The initial inflammation of the joints is followed by synovitis, arthritis, and cartilage destruction, fibrous and later bony ankylosis. The joints commonly affected are SI joints, spine, hip, and knee and manubrium sterni.

Clinical Features

Patient usually complains of early morning stiffness and pain in the back. The pain is worst at night and relieved after some activity. On examination patient has a stiff spine. Tests for sacroiliac joint involvement are positive.

Cervical spine involvement is tested by asking the patient to touch the wall with the back of the head without raising his or her chin (Fleche's test).

Thoracic Spine Involvement: If the chest expansion is less than 5 cm, involvement of thoracic spine is suspected.

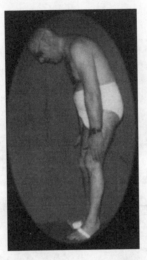

Fig. 5.34: Ankylosing spondylitis

RHEUMATOID ARTHRITIS

This has been described earlier. Orthopedic deformities of the hand (rheumatoid hand) the following are some of the very common deformities seen in the hand.

a. *Symmetrical peripheral joint swelling* of metacarpophalangeal and interphalangeal joints.

b. *Ulnar deviation* of the hand is due to rupture of the collateral ligaments at the metacarpophalangeal joints, which enables the extensor tendons to slip from their grooves towards the ulnar side.

c. *Boutonnière deformity* is due to the rupture of central extensor expansion of the fingers resulting in flexion at the PIP joint.

d. *Swan neck deformity* is due to the rupture of the volar plate of the PIP joints which enables the tendons to slip towards the dorsal side. This is also known as *intrinsic plus deformity*. Here there is hyperextension of the PIP joint and flexion of the DIP joints.

e. *Trigger fingers and trigger thumb are* due to nodules over the tendons.

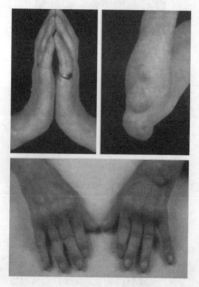

Fig. 5.35: Rheumatoid hand

GOUT

It is usually associated with hyperuricemia and may be associated with hypertension, obesity and atherosclerosis. It has an abrupt onset. Patient may complain of pain, swelling, tenderness and increased temperature of the first metatarsophalangeal joint. Frequent gouty attacks disturb the sleep. Sometimes the inflammation is so gross that it may resemble cellulitis. Attacks are provoked by surgery, trauma, etc. Mild attacks resolve spontaneously within two days, more severe attacks may last for 7 to 10 days.

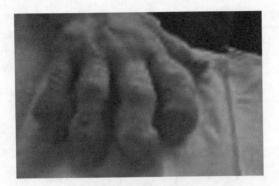

Fig. 5.36: Gout

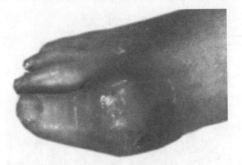

Fig. 5.37: Gout - First MTP joint affected

INFECTIVE DISORDERS

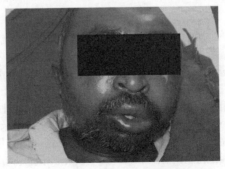

Fig. 5.38: Cellulitis of the face

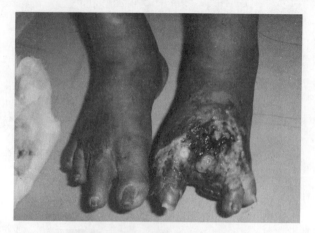

Fig. 5.39: TAO

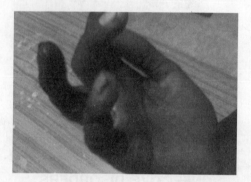

Fig. 5.40: Ischemic necrosis

LEPROSY IN ORTHOPEDICS

Leprosy is a chronic infectious disease caused by *Mycobacterium leprae*. It affects mainly the peripheral nerves and affects the skin, muscles, bones, testes and internal organs. Clinically it is characterized in early stages by hypopigmented patches, loss of cutaneous sensation, thickened nerves, and presence of acid-fast bacilli in the skin or nasal smears. *In late stages by trophic ulcers, foot-drop/claw toes , claw hand, nasal bridge collapse, loss of fingers or toes.*

Orthopedic Affections in Leprosy

Ankle and foot: Every kind of deformity is seen in the foot. Deformity is gross, because patient continues to use the foot due to loss of sensations. Ankle is rarely affected in this disease. In leprosy due to loss of sensation, there is absence of warning pain because of which, there is injury. Secondary infection following the injury is common.

Foot drop: This is one of the very common complications encountered in leprosy. It is seen in 2 percent of the cases. Common peroneal nerve is more commonly involved. Usually it is completely damaged, sometimes only deep peroneal or superficial branch is involved and occasionally only external hallucis longus muscle is involved.

Plantar ulcers: This is the other important foot complication in leprosy. It is also known as trophic ulcers due to neurological deficit. It has a spontaneous onset, it is painless, persists, and recurs. Healing process is not defective. Recurrent ulceration causes progressive destruction of the skeleton.

Sites plantar ulcers are commonly seen over the ball of feet especially first metatarsal, and heel and tips of the fingers.

Affections of the hand in leprosy: The following are the common hand deformities encountered in leprosy.

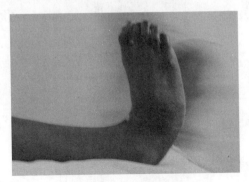

Fig. 5.41: Leprosy foot

1. *Ulnar claw hand* is due to affection of ulnar nerve at the elbow.
2. *Total claw hand* is due to affection of ulnar nerve at elbow and median nerve at the wrist.
3. *Triple nerve palsy* the following nerves are affected: ulnar nerve at the elbow, median nerve at the wrist and radial nerve at the spiral groove.

KYPHOSIS

It is defined as increase in normal posterior convexity of the thoracic spine and is referred to as 'hyper kyphosis'.

Types

Knuckle Prominence of single spinous process indicating collapse of single vertebra, e.g. TB spine/Kummel's disease, etc.

Angular 2–3 vertebral body is collapsed, e.g. late stage of TB, secondary carcinoma, etc.

Round several vertebrae are involved and hence gives a round appearance, e.g. in children—Scheuermann's disease, in old age—senile kyphosis.

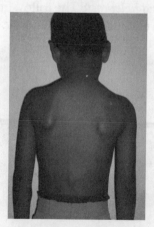

Fig. 5.42: Gibbus (knuckle type)

Methods of Examination

Look from the side and note if the thoracic curvature is regular, now determine if the kyphosis is mobile or fixed by asking the patient to bend forwards and observe for the disappearance of the deformity.

TRAUMATIC CASES

Open fracture is a surgical emergency and presents as a problem which is much more difficult than closed fractures. It is defined as a *fracture which communicates with the external atmosphere due to break in the soft tissue cover.*

Management Principles: Aims of treatment

- To convert a contaminated wound into a clean wound and thus help to convert an open fracture into a closed one.
- To establish union in a good position.
- To prevent pyogenic and clostridial infections.

Considerations

1. First priority is to stabilize the general condition of the patient as the patient is usually in shock. This consists of resuscitation, blood transfusion, intravenous fluids, antibiotics, oxygen administration, etc.
2. To keep the wound covered with proper sterile bandages till patient is ready for surgery.
3. Open fractures are surgical emergencies and surgery is to be done *as soon as the patient is fit.*
4. Proper splintage by means of external fixators.
5. ATS and AGGS to be given to avoid fatal complications like tetanus and gas gangrene.

Treatment Plan

After stabilizing the general condition of the patient, surgical debridement is planned under strict aseptic measures in major operation theaters.

External fixators are used to fix the fracture fragment after debridement. Plaster of Paris and internal fixation devices have little and controversial role in the fracture management of compound fractures. External fixator's help to stabilize fracture fragments, allow daily wound inspection and dressing, permit procedures like skin grafting, etc. to cover the wound, allow soft tissues to heal apart from providing early mobilization. In open tibial fracture, external fixator can be safely exchanged to internal fixation within 3 weeks with only 5 percent incidence of deep infection.

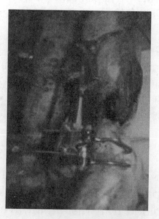

Fig. 5.43: Compound fracture tibia with external fixation

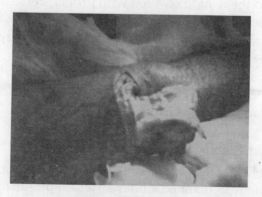

Fig. 5.44: Compound injuries

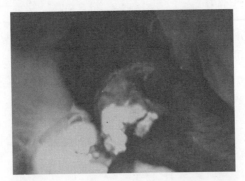

Fig. 5.45: Compound injuries—another view

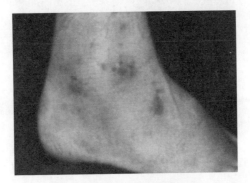

Fig. 5.46: Lateral ankle sprain

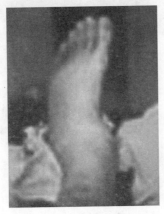

Fig. 5.47: Lateral ankle dislocation

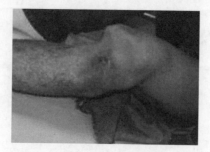

Fig. 5.48: Lateral knee dislocation

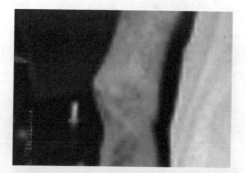

Fig. 5.49: Posterior ankle dislocation

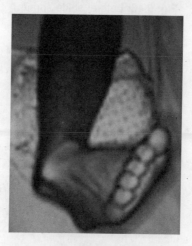

Fig. 5.50: Subtalar dislocation

AMPUTATION STUMPS

Amputation is defined as removal of the limb through a part of a bone. Disarticulation is the removal of the limb through a joint.

Limbs Eighty-five percent is through the lower limbs, 15 per cent is through the upper limbs. Injuries leading to amputations are the ones, which are severe and leave the limbs badly mutilated. High speed RTA's, major falls, and crushing injuries due to industrial or agricultural accidents spell unmitigated disaster to the limbs making amputation a logical solution. However, in children, congenital anomalies and in the elderly, peripheral vascular disease is the common causes of amputations.

Closed Amputation

This is done most of the times as an elective procedure and may be above knee or below knee, above elbow and below elbow, etc. In this, the skin is closed primarily after amputation.

Open Amputations (Guillotine Operation)

In this type of amputation the skin is not closed primarily and later it is followed by any one of the closure methods like secondary closure, reamputation, revision amputation or plastic repair depending upon the prevailing local situations.

Amputation Levels

Upper limbs Various levels of amputation at the upper limbs.
- Shoulder disarticulation
- Short above elbow
- Standard above elbow
- Elbow disarticulation
- Very short below elbow
- Medium below elbow
- Long below elbow.

Lower limbs various levels of amputations at the lower limbs are:

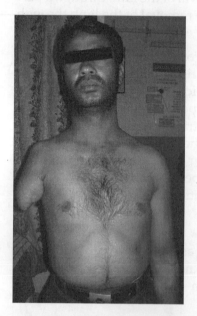

Fig. 5.51: View from the front

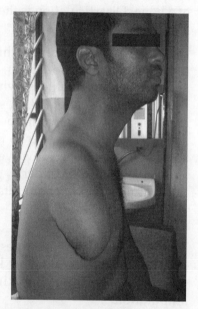

Fig. 5.52: View from the sides

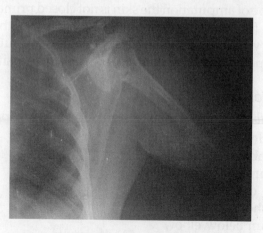

Fig. 5.53: X-ray of the stump

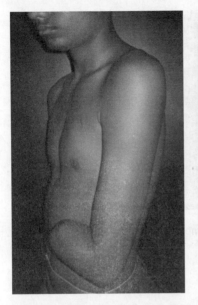

Fig. 5.54a: Below elbow amputation

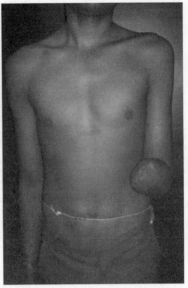

Fig. 5.54b: Below elbow amputation

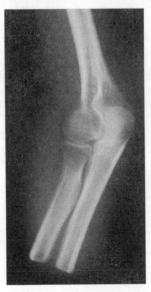

Fig. 5.54c: Below elbow amputation

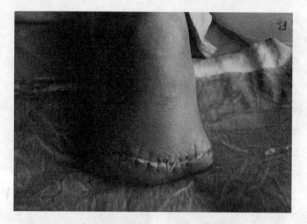

Fig. 5.55: BK amputation stump

- Hip disarticulation
- Very short above knee
- Short above knee
- Medium above knee
- Long above knee
- Very long above knee
- Knee disarticulation
- Very short below knee
- Short and below knee.

Index

Clinical Notes

Clinical Notes

Clinical Notes

Clinical Notes

Clinical Notes

Clinical Notes

Clinical Notes

Clinical Notes